The Letters of Audre Lorde and Pat Parker 1974 - 1989

Introduction by Mecca Jamilah Sullivan
Edited by Julie R. Enszer

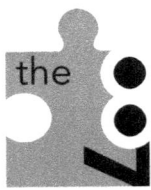

Published 2024 by the87press

The 87 Press LTD

87 Stonecot Hill

Sutton

Surrey

SM3 9HJ

www.the87press.co.uk

Copyright © *The Letters of Audre Lorde and Pat Parker 1974 – 1989*, edited by Julie R. Enszer.

Letters of Pat Parker copyright © 2018, 2024 by Anastasia Dunham-Parker-Brady. All rights reserved.

Letters of Audre Lorde copyright © 2018, 2024 by the Audre Lorde Estate. All rights reserved.

Introduction copyright © 2018, 2024 by Mecca Jamilah Sullivan.

All rights reserved.

First published in the USA in 2018 by Sinister Wisdom, Inc.

The moral right of the authors have been asserted in accordance with the Copyright, Designs and Patents Act 1988

ISBN: 978-1-0686446-1-0

Printed and bound by CPI Group (UK) Ltd, Croydon, CR0 4YY
Cover Photograph Credit: Susan Fleischmann, © 1981, 2024
Design: Stanislava Stoilova [www.sdesign.graphics]

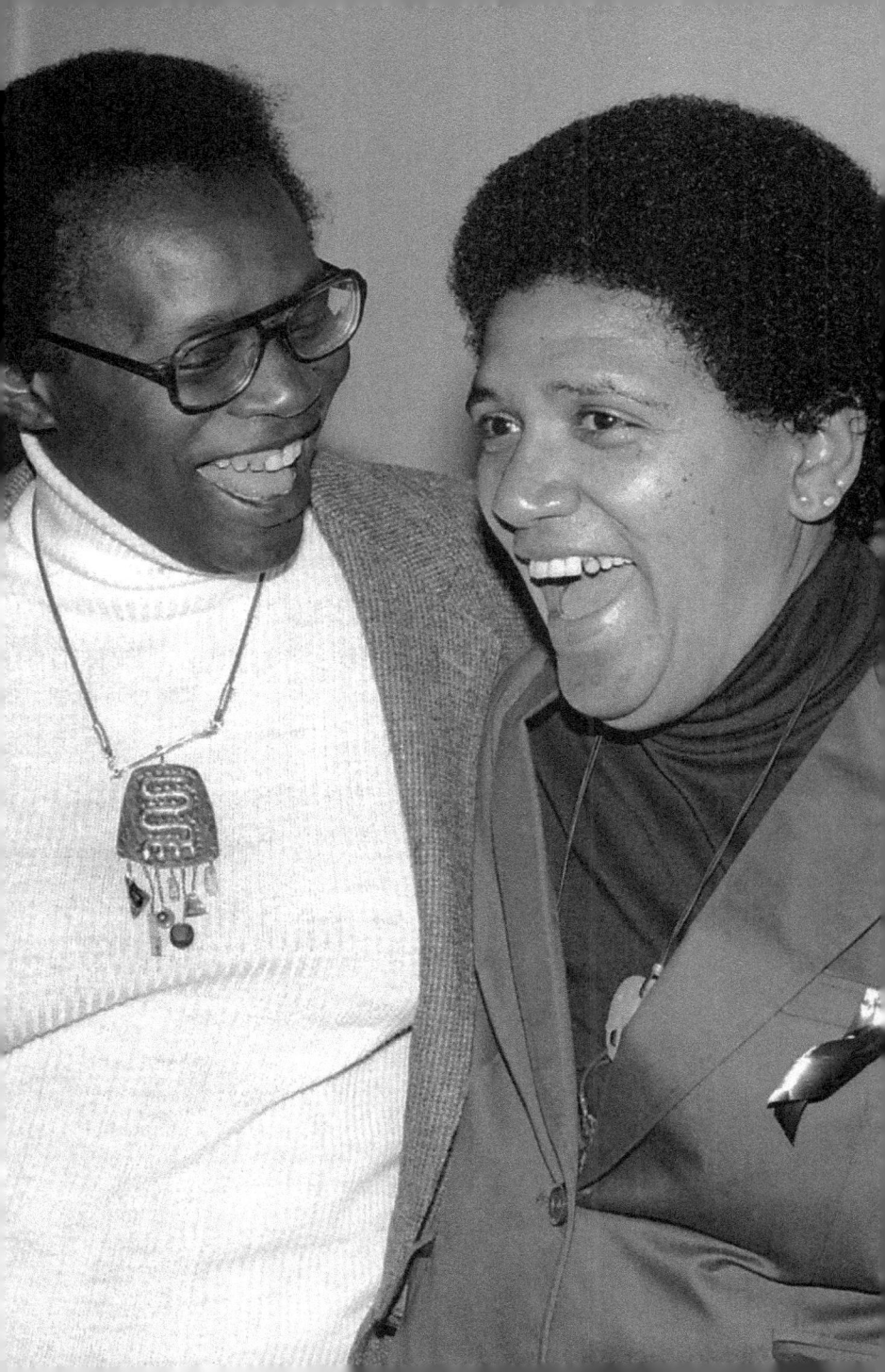

For the children and grandchildren of
Pat Parker and Audre Lorde

Contents

Introduction by Mecca Jamilah Sullivan	1
Letters	15
Editor's Note	105
Acknowledgements	107
Audre Lorde Partial Bibliography	109
Pat Parker Partial Bibliography	111

Introduction

"I think you changed the world": Black Lesbian Feminism in Love and Letters

There were poems in her mouth, on the tables, in the refrigerator, under the bed, and in the way she cast about the apartment, searching for—not answers—but rather, unexpressable questions. We were both Black; we were both Lesbians; we were both poets in a very white, straight, male world, and we sat up all night trading poems.

—Audre Lorde, Foreword to Pat Parker's
Movement in Black (1978)

> Now this woman
> sits in my house
> reads
>   no devours
>   my words.
>
> No comment.
>
> Just
> clicking and um-humming
> then has the nerve
> to say I write good but
> not enough.
>
> *Push more*
> *take the harder road.*

Who is this woman?

—Pat Parker, "For Audre" (1986)

Reading writers' letters is the best kind of eavesdropping. It brings the rush and sweetness of hidden listening—the secret drinking-in of voices children thrive on, clinging to doorways, palms slick, ready to learn what they have yearned and yearned to know. The hiddenness somehow makes the listening better: these words are not meant for *us* but for a world before and beyond us, and so each syllable is a gem. The words demand we reach for them and that we grow in the reaching.

Whether we are (as I am) the grown-up black/queer/women/writer versions of little black girls eavesdropping on our mothers and aunties at the kitchen table, or are queer, or women, or feminist in some other way, this stunning volume of letters between Audre Lorde and Pat Parker carries that breathlessness of urgent listening, the thrill that sparks when learning is both demanding and deeply sweet.

As poets, writers, activists, and thinkers, Lorde and Parker's immense contributions to feminist, black, lesbian, queer, and American literary culture cannot be overstated. Their combined oeuvres include over twenty poetry collections and non-fiction monographs; dozens of published poems, essays, and lectures; and several short stories, plays, performance pieces and mixed-genre works[1]. With these works—and with their activism and teaching—Lorde and Parker made foundational contributions to feminist discourses of the 1970s and 1980s and offered incisive critiques of gender,

---

[1] See Audre Lorde, *Zami: A New Spelling of My Name* (Freedom, CA: Crossing Press, 1982). See also Pat Parker, "Two Plays" and "Prose" in *The Collected Works of Pat Parker.* Ed. Julie R. Enszer, (Dover, FL: A Midsummer Night's Press and Sinister Wisdom, 2016).

sexuality, race, class, and power around which black feminism takes its shape today.

Lorde and Parker sit at opposite points of the kitchen tables—real and figurative—around which my black queer feminist literary politic has taken shape. I encountered Lorde in the late 1990s as a teenager in high school—Hunter High School, which Lorde had also attended some forty-five years earlier. I discovered her autobiographical coming-of-age "biomythography," *Zami*, and immediately felt what would become a familiar mix of rapture and rage. Like many of us, I was awed at the precision with which she articulated black lesbian feminist life, a life that was just beginning to unfold for me. I was grateful for the intimate sense of history she offered, the proof she gave of a black queer political and literary past that I needed badly without knowing I needed it. I was also enraged that I had not learned about her before, particularly as I had also grown up on the same Harlem block she describes in *Zami* (far across town from Hunter), and had attended the Catholic church where she went to grade school. That something so necessary as her work could be erased from all these spaces—the coinciding spaces of school, home, and spirit—infuriated me. That anger needled deeper years later when I finally learned of Pat Parker through Alexis De Veaux's pathbreaking *Warrior Poet: A Biograpy of Audre Lorde*.[2] In *Warrior Poet*, De Veaux offers an extremely moving and important picture of the friendship between Lorde and Parker. By that time, I had recently finished my B.A. in Afro-American Studies at a women's college and was applying to Ph.D. programs to study gender and sexuality in black women's literature. I was both baffled and incensed by this long path to Parker, whose legacy has been even more silenced than Lorde's, even in many feminist circles.

---

[2]De Veaux, Alexis, *Warrior Poet: A Biography of Audre Lorde* (New York: W.W. Norton & Co., 2004).

The letters gathered here fill those silences. Expertly edited by Julie R. Enszer and culled from the archives of Spelman College and the Schlesinger Library at the Radcliffe Institute for Advanced Study, the dialogue we overhear in these pages traces not only the shared processes of thought and questioning through which these writers' works come into being, but also maps the creation story of the black feminist literary practice and politics that, for many of us, shapes the work we do today. In these letters, we overhear a history of collaborative self-authorship and self-authorization, a process of survival that comprises humor, anger, tension and tenderness as these women write themselves—and us—into a black feminist future.

Sent between 1974 and 1988 (the year before Parker's death and four years before Lorde's) these letters steep us in the complex intellectual and political intimacy and *work* involved in creating what we now term "Black Feminist Literature." The letters offer a breathtaking narrative history of some of the many important feminist publications, organizations, events and activist groups of the 1970s and 1980s that shaped their world and have set the stage for contemporary black feminist, feminist, lesbian, and queer arts and activism, including: *Conditions*, *Amazon Quarterly*, Gente, Diana Press, Shameless Hussy Press, *Off Our Backs*, FESTAC (the Second World African Festival of the Arts, held in Lagos in 1977), and others. Enszer's detailed and thorough notes offer fantastically rich context for this history. We witness as Lorde and Parker navigate not only the structural and organizational dynamics of the feminist scene, but also work through its most pressing intellectual and political questions, including the need for black feminist organizing, the responsibilities and ethics of feminist publishing, the racism within white feminist communities, and the possibilities of a global black feminist praxis, pushing one-another's thinking forward, and working through the key ideas on which our current black feminist politics rely. Take, for example, Parker's April 29th, 1980 letter to Lorde, in which she writes:

> I feel now is the time for people to understand and implement coalition politics; that now is the time for an organization that addresses itself not only to the needs of Black people in this country but to have a global perspective and understand our connection with other third world countries... not only are we anti-sexist, racist, fascist, but also we are anti-imperialist and we are opposed to the stand that this country has taken in its dealings with other countries in the world particularly third world countries.[3]

Here and in their other work, Parker and Lorde imagine a black feminism both focused and capacious enough to understand the interrelatedness of multiple power structures, and to address the interdependence of racism, sexism, heterosexism, classism as key parts of a matrix of power shaping the conditions of black women's lives, extending the Combahee River Collective's groundbreaking 1977 "Black Feminist Statement," and anticipating the work of legal theorist Kimberlé Crenshaw, who coins the term "intersectionality" to describe this concept in 1989.[4] Parker's interest in using black feminism to understand and critique US actions in Iran articulate a crucial vision for a global intersectionality

---

[3] Audre Lorde and Pat Parker, *The Letters of Audre Lorde and Pat Parker, 1974 – 1989*, edited by Julie R. Enszer (the87press, 2024), 41.

[4] See The Combahee River Collective, "Black Feminist Statement" in *Home Girls: A Black Feminist Anthology*. Ed. Barbara Smith (New York: Kitchen Table / Women of Color Press, 1983), 264-74. See also Kimberlé Crenshaw, "Demarginalizing the Intersection of Race and Sex: A Black Feminist Critique of Antidiscrimination Doctrine, Feminist Theory and Antiracist Politics." *University of Chicago Legal Forum* (1989): 139-167.

arguably more expansive than many of those that circulate in popular feminist media and academic discourse today.

As much as these letters shape and historicize the building of a black feminist literary politics in the twentieth century, eavesdropping on this conversation also makes clear the very personal stakes involved in the building of a black feminist literary politics. Parker's and Lorde's theoretical heavy-lifting takes place alongside discussions of creative insecurities, the art of self-promotion, the impulse to procrastinate, and the very real daily business of paying the bills and making ends meet. On most of these points, Lorde assumes the role of Parker's mentor, offering advice with a blend of toughness and tenderness that demonstrates the urgency of the black feminist literary project in the 70s and 80s, and the key role that interpersonal networks play in sustaining that project amid shifting and sometimes precarious institutional structures. In an undated letter to Parker, Lorde warns:

> Now. I wish I could have this letter self-destruct like *Mission Impossible*, but I can't, so don't please leave it lying around. The thing about these Poetry in the Schools gig is this: get in there, give the kids what you can (and from you that's a lot) make a lot of bread, which is possible if you play it right, but don't stay around too long. AND DON'T TRUST ANYONE IN IT. [...] Consider seriously what I've just said, but keep your mouth shut about it to EVERYBODY, or both our asses are liable to wind up in the street.[5]

Yet, even in this high-stakes environment, tenderness persists reciprocally at the conversation's core, pushing both women forward not only in their thinking and work but also in their

---

[5] *The Letters of Audre Lorde and Pat Parker*, 19.

lives. When Parker apologizes for asking Lorde to "retrace... a lot of familiar ground," in their letters about breast cancer (which ultimately claimed both women's lives) Lorde replies:

> Listen, love... it's like being in a relationship with a beloved part of my own self. It's always been so difficult to love you from afar, and so costly to come in close, I put a lot of the stuff I learned about you and me into EYE TO EYE.[6]

This is one of these letters' many delights for eavesdroppers who love black feminist literature: they offer into nuanced insight into the complex inner worlds of these two writers and the intimacy between them. As De Veaux notes, this was a relationship of both love and tension, one in which Lorde took "a bullheaded delight in playing the big sister role" while "Parker's refusal to behave like a doting fan, or treat... Lorde as anything but a peer, confounded her; yet it was also the deeper reason Lorde respected Parker."[7] We see these tensions play out in the letters, but we also see them balanced with a surprising humor and playfulness not often associated with either woman and especially not with the famously serious and self-possessed Lorde. For example, in an undated 1975 postcard to Parker we see a "hand drawn drawing of a rabbit by Lorde with the words: WHAT'S UP DOC?" Likewise, in closing the February 16, 1986 letter with which she sends Lorde the poem "For Audre," Parker writes: "Going to close this up. Please take care of yourself and give my love to Frances. I look forward to seeing her. Love, Pat P.S. How do you cook beets?"

---

[6]Ibid., 77.

[7]De Veaux, 287, 168.

These moments of levity are not simply footnotes to the larger project of black lesbian feminist political praxis; they echo an understanding crucial to both Lorde's and Parker's work: that the rich terrains of intimacy are key sites of feminist praxis. The letters read, at times, as a dialogue of girlfriends, sounding in some ways like the familiar banter of the characters in Parker's plays—smart and melodic, with a poetic efficiency, and again, always available to a quick departure into humorous critique of racism, sexism, homophobia, and power. In her July 24, 1975 letter to Lorde, for example, Parker writes:

> Have also got to put myself on a diet. Gained a great deal of weight. Feel like I'm dragging about triplets. Can't afford to ruin my image as a sex symbol, right? I think someone in my neighborhood is expressing their opinion of our sexual preferences. I've had three flat tires this week. (27)

The letters also bespeak intimacy in its most familiar senses: Parker shares her coming out story with Lorde, who regards Parker as the first out black lesbian she ever met—an experience she describes in her Foreword to Parker's poetry collection *Movement in Black*, excerpted above (DeVeaux, *Warrior Poet* 169). Lorde likewise often sends money with her letters, offering various explanations for the gifts. Yet, perhaps unsurprisingly, the gifts we see exchanged most frequently here are those of support and advice. It is this kind of generosity we see at play when Parker reveals, in the July 25, 1975 letter, that she is considering going back to college, and Lorde replies, emphatically: "learn what you want and don't be AFRAID."[8]

This real-time dialogue on the nuts and bolts of black feminist writing may be one of the greatest pleasures available

---

[8]*The Letters of Audre Lorde and Pat Parker,* 36.

to the eavesdropper here. Both writers refer to (and sometimes outright quote) their own now well-known works, and we observe as they reflect on their own poetics and craft, both in the content of their conversation and in the form of the letters themselves. Over the course of their friendship, Lorde offers Parker ample advice on her poems, as Parker's "For Audre," suggests. And, especially in the earlier letters, we hear Lorde teach Parker to craft the arc of her own career with the careful self-awareness of a master plot architect. In her January 18, 1975 letter to Lorde, we see Parker integrate this reflection on craft into the conversation's poetics, beginning the letter with an epigraph:

> Once upon a time there was this woman named Audre and she met this woman named Pat. And she faithfully wrote her a letter. And for a long time she waited, but there was no answer[...] And the moral of this dyke tale, children, is that Pat Parker is alive and well but just a little more crazier. THE END.[9]

It is fitting that these two women, though widely known as poets, should return so often to storytelling modes, both as a metaphor and as a tool for professional and political movement. After all, both women used writing as a tool for exploring intersectional multiplicity, writing in and across the genres of poetry, prose fiction, drama, criticism, performance, and scholarship, often expanding, questioning, and reimagining each as she went. Parker comments on this directly in her January 4, 1988 letter to Lorde, in which she remarks:

> It's amazing to me how you are world renowned as a poet, women falling all over themselves to get next to you, and I always feel closer to you through your

---

[9]Ibid., 21.

prose. There's a vulnerability there that makes me want to gather you in my arms and hold you.[10]

For these women, writing across genres means not only more expansive expressions of black feminist political life, but also more and deeper points of access to each other. Together, they are creative writers and scholars, novelists and theorists, dramatists and poets and performers and educators and many things in between. Reading from our contemporary moment, these careers may be somewhat difficult to imagine, particularly for those ensconced in the academic world of disciplines, departments, and fiercely guarded fields (social sciences over here, literary studies over there, black studies, women's studies, and LGBT studies somewhere in-between, and creative writing way down the street, with poets, playwrights and fiction writers each in their own mysterious silos). This is not the way Lorde and Parker wrote. Their deliberate movements across genres offer hope and instruction: they are not writing for institutions; they are writing for the record, for power and posterity, for their own paychecks and also for the many black queer women's lives that breathe invisibly in futures beyond them.[11]

This emphasis on a black feminist futurity is palpable throughout the letters, particularly toward the conversation's end. Both Lorde and Parker were thoughtful teachers,

---

[10]Ibid., 75.

[11]Throughout the letters, we also gain fascinating insight into how technology shapes their engagements with futurity, a conversation subtheme that also becomes a space for humor and intimacy. Parker teases the older Lorde for using a typewriter (rather than a word processor), and Lorde later offers, in mock defensiveness, "Not only have I become computer literate (are you ready for this language) but even computer artistic!" and "I do have a modem." Assimilating computer information technology and other technological advancements also becomes a way to help each other further their work: Lorde asks Parker for advice on computer brands and word processing programs, while Parker offers to send VHS videotapes of Baldwin, asking "Do you have a VCR in your house?"

deliberate about their pedagogy and invested in teaching as a political tool inextricable from their own writing.[12] After a workshop for children at the National Women's Music Festival in Bloomington, IN—a trip that inspired what later became an important essay, "Poetry at Women's Music Festivals: Oil and Water," Parker reflects: "I'd forgotten, how much I enjoyed working with kids in schools" (59).[13] Likewise, Lorde describes a reading she and poet Cheryl Clarke gave to benefit a student-run lesbian magazine, remarking: "…it gave me an enormous charge to feel what such an event could mean just in terms of change and the world's story and us, etc. and looking at their wonderful young faces? I felt very blessed to be who I am and where I was and a part of it all."[14]

The letters' attunement to the future amplifies toward the end of this collection, as Parker and Lorde support one-another through the fear, pain, and uncertainty of coping with breast cancer. In these exchanges, they offer lucid, haunting insights about black women and death, a theme that unearths questions of race, gender, economics, healthcare, bodily rights and autonomy deeply relevant today. Discussing the choice and between chemotherapy and holistic approaches to cancer treatment in her January 4th, 1988 letter, Parker observes: "If I live five years from now, both sides can claim a victory of sorts. And if I die, then both can blame the other for my demise. Or more likely, I'll be blamed,"[15] articulating nearly perfectly the

---

[12] Lorde wrote frequently about the importance of teaching for her political and creative work. See Audre Lorde, "Poet as Teacher—Human as Poet—Teacher as Human," in *I Am Your Sister: Collected and Unpublished Writings of Audre Lorde.*, Ed. Rudolph P. Byrd, Johnnetta Betsch Cole, and Beverely Guy-Sheftall. (London: Oxford University Press, 2011), 182-183.

[13] See Pat Parker, "Poetry at Women's Music Festivals: Oil and Water," in *The Collected Works of Pat Parker*. Ed. Julie R. Enszer (New York: A Midsummer Night's Press and Sinister Wisdom, 2016).

[14] *The Letters of Audre Lorde and Pat Parker,* 53.

[15] Ibid., 69.

multiple conundrums of race, gender, class, and embodiment that shape the medical industrial complex today.

Even as Lorde and Parker struggle together to come to terms with mortality and illness, we hear how this shared coping not only gives them life (as the queer children say today), but also give the love between them a new kind of living, one keenly attentive to the immediate necessity of intimate connection for both bodily survival and intellectual legacy. In their last letters, we witness the roaring depth of their shared vulnerability to mortality, which we also hear in Parker's "For Audre": "I kissed the space where/ your right breast had been/ ran my tongue over your body/ to lick away your fear/ to lick away my fear."

In these letters, we hear all this take shape in ink—the fear, the space, the toughness, the bodies licking away—as these two luminary black lesbian women teach themselves and each other the lessons we all need to learn, then, now, and for the future. This is nowhere clearer than in Lorde's December 6th, 1985 advice to Parker:

> Things you must be aware of right now—
>
> A year seems like a lot of time now at this end—it isn't.... Don't lose your sense of urgency on the one hand, on the other, don't be too hard on yourself—or expect too much.
> Beware the terror of not producing.
> Beware the urge to justify your decision.
> Watch out for the kitchen sink and the plumbing and that painting that always needed being done.
> But remember the body needs to create to.
> Beware feeling you're not good enough to deserve it
> Beware feeling you're too good to need it
> Beware all the hatred you've stored up inside

you, and the locks on your tender places.[16]

Ultimately, these letters teach us more of what we've needed to know about these two women whose works are as illuminating and as needed today as they were during their lifetimes. Yet they also give us lessons for our own work, and our own living. Among these lessons are so many gems that echo and extend the political contributions of their published writing, for which we cherish them now: lessons about creating oneself, honoring one's work as crucial legacy, battling tenderly with and for community, and using words to imagine new futures. As Lorde puts it in her February 6th, 1988 letter: "The fact that we're writing these letters to each other is a triumph, Pat, I feel it and want you to feel it too. You been doing what you came to do, sweetheart, and I think you changed the world."

In this context of urgent teaching and tenderness aflame, it is, in a way, surprising that Parker ends one section of her poem "For Audre" not with triumph, but with a note of apology. Parker writes:

> I felt jealous wanted to be near you
> and to hold you
> and to sing you songs
> to say I love you
> you are not alone
> then I felt guilt for all the unsent letters
> for all the unwritten poems
> for all the 'dead air.'

As black girls, queer kids, trans folks, womanists, lesbians, feminists, and radicals in-becoming, as we read this book, we know that the air between these letters is anything but dead.

---

[16] Ibid., 54.

It breathes life and *lives*—lives lived fiercely and documented generously so that we may keep them going.

Mecca Jamilah Sullivan, PhD
February 2018

October 12, 1974

Dear Pat:

Warmth from a cold place[1] to you and Ann.[2] It was so good to see you again, and to meet Ann. I hope things are going well with you both.

Having come up for air after the deluge of work descending upon me on my return, I find, in rapid and devastating succession that: 1) my copy of Paper Trip upon which I wrote your address is missing, so I've got to scurry about and find it again[3] 2) you're in the forthcoming Directory of American Poets, not the last, so that doesn't help me either, 3) you managed not to give me a copy of your new long poem, which was pretty slick of you but not very nice, since I asked you at least twice,[4] and 4) you have not yet written to Galen Williams,[5] which is a mistake. Get it together, lady. Of course it's not REALLY important on the cosmic scale of things: we both know it, but like every other kind of grease, it helps to keep the kinks at least manageable and I know you know what I mean.

---

[1] Lorde's letterhead indicates that she was writing from her home on St. Paul's Avenue in Staten Island.

[2] Ann Bernard was Parker's lover in October 1974.

[3] "Paper Trip" was a small pamphlet first published in Iowa City by The People's Press with the subtitle, "the how and why's of getting false I.D.'s: a manual on how to get false I.D.'s for draft evaders, military deserters, fugitives from the "law", underage people, runaways and just plain people."

[4] It is unclear which long poem Lorde is referencing, but Parker was possibly working on either "Movement in Black" (95) or "Womanslaughter" (149) in 1974 (Dover, FL: *The Complete Poems of Pat Parker*, Sinister Wisdom/A Midsummer Night's Press, 2016).

[5] Galen Williams was the director of the Poetry Center at the 92nd Street Y in New York City from 1961 until 1970 and then the founder of Poets & Writers. Lorde encouraged Parker to write to Williams about the Poets in Schools program (discussed later in the correspondence.)

Anyway, spoke to Galen this morning about you and she was moderately unhelpful, although she does know your name and *Child of Myself*.[6] For readings, she suggests you write to the people on the lists I'm sending you, using my name, telling them you plan to be in the area during such-and-such a time, and would be interested in—or rather, are available for—a reading.

Now what this means of course is that you must decide on a time—and I suggest sometime next spring, because these places get their money in April—when you can come East. In addition, get the names of women's groups and bookshops here (I'm working on compiling that for you, but maybe Alice can help, there) and send the same kind of letter to them. At best, you won't hear from more than ¼ of them, but that's a start. If you're interested, that is. It does mean work.

Also, please send me some poems for *Amazon Quarterly*.[7] I'm also very interested in knowing what's happening with the Third World Women's group[8] you're working with. What's happening with the writing workshops? Has it gotten off the ground?

Give my love to Ann, and write me soon, or I'll haunt you.

Love,
Audre

P.S. In your letter, don't forget to include the names of your books and other publications, and that you're a Black Feminist Poet. The checks are the ones I particularly suggest.[9]

---

[6] Shameless Hussy Press, operated by alta in San Lorenzo, CA, first published Parker's chapbook, *Child of Myself*, in 1971; in 1972, Parker joined the Women's Press Collective in Oakland, CA and the Women's Press Collective released two editions of *Child of Myself*, one in 1972 and one in 1974.

[7] Lorde was the poetry editor for *Amazon Quarterly*, often abbreviated as *AQ*.

[8] Gente is the group Lorde references here; for more information about Gente see note 12.

[9] I have not seen a copy of the list that apparently accompanied this letter.

SET II

Pat: I particularly want the long poem and the poem to white women who want to be friendly (I can't remember the exact title)[10] for *AQ*.[11] AND FAST. We go to press on the 20th. Can you make it?

---

[10]Lorde refers to Parker's poem "For the white person who wants to know how to be my friend" (*The Complete Works of Pat Parker*, 76.)

[11]*Amazon Quarterly*.

[undated, typewritten letter]

Dear Pat:

Thanks for the poems. Too late for this issue: I'll let you know when we can run them. So good to hear from you, and about Ann. Tell her good luck from me, and to really wow them, which I know she will. About Felicia: please help her in any way you can. She's my "baby sister," ask her about it sometime. But the two of you are like pieces of my own flesh far away, and that's a kind of bond. She needs Gente.[12] She also needs you.

Great about Poetry in the Schools program. It wasn't too difficult, but I want to tell you some things about it. First, I'm sending you herewith a Newsletter from T&W,[13] a NY outfit that I worked with some years ago, and which has a lot of good stuff in it on possible approaches. Check out the diaries from SF State I've checked, and also send for the Whole Word Cat[14]...

---

[12]Gente was a women of color organization in the San Francisco/Oakland Bay Area. Parker helped found and nourish the organization over many years and participated and lead many of its activities. In July 1974, *Lesbian Tide* described "Gente" as "an all Third World Lesbian softball team, the first of its kind that we know of." At the time, the team included twenty-five women "from nearly every nationality that is a part of the growing Liberation movement of Third World people. . .Raza (Chicana and Puerta Rican), Black (including a sister from the West Indies), Native American and Asian American." The description continued, "They are a mixture of folks from factory teams and folks with degrees. Bread to start and sustain the team was raised from a woman's corporation and from a fund-raising dance they threw themselves. They have no sponsor, they provide their own spark." Gente also performed as the Gente Gospelaires under the direction of Linda Tillery, vocalist, producer, percussionist, and cultural historian. The Gente Gospelaires sang at community events and fundraisers (see Parker's reference to singing with the group on page 36).

[13]Teachers & Writers.

[14]Teachers & Writers published *The Whole Word Catalogue*, edited by Rosellen Brown, Marvin Hoffman, Marvin Kushner, Phillip Lopate, and Sheila Murphy; it was "a compendium of writing ideas and activities culled from our magazines and from writers' journals." Teachers & Writers sold over 100,000 copies of the book.

it's very fine. (If you can) Now. I wish I could have this letter self-destruct like *Mission Impossible*, but I can't, so don't please leave it lying around. The thing about these Poetry in Schools gigs is this: get in there, give the kids what you can (and from you that's a lot) make a lot of bread, which is possible if you play it right, but don't stay around too long. AND DON'T TRUST ANYONE IN IT. Play it cool, keep your mouth shut when you're not poeting, and don't get <u>too</u> buddy-bud with the poets you work with. Protect yourself <u>at all times,</u> and the kids, if you can. I believe it's a testing-ground for a lot of things, none of which you need to be involved with. I'm saying these things to you because I trust you, which is why I made the original connection. Use it, and then get out. And remember, nothing connected with the National Endowment for the Arts (NEA) which funds it, and funds a lot of programs you'll probably be getting more and more involved with in the future; NOTHING connected with the NEA is only what it seems to be on the surface.

Consider seriously what I've just said, but keep your mouth shut about it to EVERYBODY, or both our asses are liable to wind up in the street. (Not that they both haven't been there before, honey, but why press a good thing...) And the kids <u>do</u> need what you have to give them.

Sounds good about GENTE. There's a couple hundred dollars (5 to be exact) floating around I think the group could use.[15] If you're interested, after you all decide about incorporating and that jazz, please send me a letter, sort of formal-like, telling about the group and dealing with the following: <u>Purpose; Composition; Programs; Future Plans; and Goals.</u> By formal-like I mean keep in mind it's not for my eyes only. Two other women poets involved—very fine people but more or less straight. If, on the other hand, you decide not to bother, or it's not worth it, let me know right away and I'll stop

---

[15]Lorde facilitated a grant to Gente.

sitting on the dough, because I've had Gente in my mind since we first talked about it.

Of course you can read my poems to the women. But do something for me: find out if any of them are writing themselves, and ask them to send their poems to me for consideration to publish in *Amazon Quarterly*. I want to do a POETRY FOR PRISON issue. Kiss Ann for me, and you stay strong and beautiful. I love you.

Audre

P.S. I'm sending the Newsletter under separate cover. Please let me know if this letter gets to you okay and in good condition. And next time, seal your envelopes: the enclosed check is for stamps and Bazooka Bubble Gum, if they make it out your way. Happy St. Toad's Day![16]

---

[16] The post-script was added at the top of the one page letter; it has been moved to the end for reading convenience.

January 18, 1975

Once upon a time there was this woman named Audre and she met this woman named Pat. And she faithfully wrote her a letter. And for a long time she waited, but there was no answer. So Audre who knew that Pat lived in the land of the poet-killers assumed that her friend must be dead: for she knew that that was the only reason Pat hadn't answered her letter. She knew that Pat wasn't one of those "lazy niggers." And one day out of the great smoggy blue a letter came and lo and behold it was from Pat and Audre rejoiced, for she knew that her friend wasn't dead, but alas she had to admit and realized that her friend was indeed a "lazy nigger." And the moral of this dyke tale, children, is that Pat Parker is alive and well but just a little more crazier.

THE END

Audre, hello

You can see what working with elementary school children has done with my brain. Just completed my ten weeks. Spent the last two weeks typing ditto masters and for a slow inaccurate typist like me that was pure hell. Even got to the point where I was willing to hire a typist, but I couldn't find one willing to take on that mess. I enjoyed it though. The kids were beautiful. And that's the last time I [am] going to try and correct an error. The teachers on the other hand were a pain in the ass. There was this constant echo saying watch your spelling children.

Gente is still going strong. There are two women working on proposals. I told the group about you and your friends. We're having our monthly business meeting tonight. Should find out how the incorporation is moving.

Haven't seen or talked to Felicia in some time. Had made a deal with her. She was supposed to sell Ann and me her bike, but she changed her mind. She said she was moving and needed more money than either of us had. I don't know where she is. Which has me a little distressed since she's got my ten-speed.

Went down to California Institute for Women. The inmates liked my poetry. The prison officials weren't so happy about it. They denied me the right to do my second reading. I did it anyway, but had to have lookouts watching for guards. Spent most of the second reading listening to their poetry. Some of which was really good. Told them to send it off to you. They seemed excited about that suggestion. The guards searched me and my briefcase. They had a woman searching me while another guard searched my briefcase. And used that opportunity to steal one of my notebooks And I wasn't sure I had brought that notebook, so I wasn't positive they had ripped it until I checked my studio when I got home. It was my working notebook, which I usually don't take to readings.

Ann's hard at work on my trip.[17] She's compiled a list of all my publications and readings for the last 5 years or so. She and Paula Wallace[18] composed a letter to send off. So now she and Wendy Cadden[19] are at work. At least that is what I'm being told. So I definitely will be out there in May.

Oh, I sent off for the Directory of American Poets for last year, but they had sold out. Now if I'm correct and am in the one for this year then I don't have to pay for this one right?

---

[17]Parker and Judy Grahn went on a cross-country trip reading poetry from June through July 1975.

[18]Paula Wallace was a photography and member of the Women's Press Collective. She learned bookselling at A Woman's Place Bookstore in Oakland, CA and with Carol Seajay founded and operated Old Wives' Tales, the feminist bookstore in San Francisco. Wallace was also the publisher of Full Circle Books in Albuquerque, NM.

[19]Wendy Cadden was a member of the Women's Press Collective and a graphic artist. Her graphic work was featured in many Women's Press Collective books.

Ann just came in and brought me the registration for the truck. The rest of this letter is being typed in a state of shock. In fact, I think I will end this and get moving. A friend of mine just had a baby boy and a broken car and I'm the unofficial chauffeur for milk, baby clothes, etc.

Just finished another poem for Ann.[20] Am including it in this letter. This is the first draft and any and all criticism will be accepted. Also tell me about the NEA fellowships.

Take care and don't take as long as I do to answer letters.

    easy,
    Pat

---

[20] Two poems for Ann are in *The Complete Works of Pat Parker*: "Poem #4 for Ann" (390) and "Poem for Ann #5" (393).

[undated – likely April 1975]

Dear Pat,[21]

When are you all coming & what're your plans? I need to know.

How are things going?

Love to you both.
Audre

---

[21]This postcard contains a hand drawing of a rabbit by Lorde with the words: WHAT'S UP DOC?

7/15 [1975]

Dear Pat

What's gone down in the past few months re *AQ* is too ugly to rehash- suffice it to say the next issue will probably be the last- at any rate it will certainly be my last.[22] I've given your two poems to the women planning the Amazon Poets Anthology & you should be hearing directly from them.[23] If this is not to your desire, tell me & I'll get them back - it's just that I wanted the women whose poems I'd intended to print in *AQ* (yours among them) to have some other option other than the gnashing of teeth.[24]

My love to you & Ann, and it's been real nice hearing from you!

Audre

AQ shouldn't have been a total loss, at least I've learned something – if only to say no in the future!

A[25]

---

[22] *Amazon Quarterly* published the last issue in March 1975.

[23] Elly Bulkin and Joan Larkin edited and published *Amazon Poetry* in 1975.

[24] Parker's poems did not appear in AQ. Joan Larkin and Elly Bulkin published the poems "Sunday" and "For Willyce" in *Amazon Poetry* (Brooklyn: Out & Out Books, 1975).

[25] This is a handwritten letter on a note pad that reads "From the desk of Audre Lorde".

July 24, 1975

Hello Audre,

That may be the last cheerful thing you'll see in this letter. Audre, please forgive my failure to write sooner. Times have been hectic and hard in these parts. Would you believe that as I was typing this letter the typewriter broke? I just spend the last ½ hour cursing out the typewriter repair company that I just finished paying $70 for fixing it a month ago. The repairman told me how to fix it on the phone, but I'll have to take it back in and have them readjust their readjustment. If there were another person in the house right now I'd probably kill them. It's about par for the course.

We got home the first week in June. The Gente Gospelaires were scheduled to sing twice that weekend. So, off I went singing. I was scheduled to read twice that weekend. I still don't know what I could have been thinking about to let Ann do that. I missed one reading. Somehow put it in my mind that I was to read at one time when was in fact an hour later. Had a softball game to play so off I went, played the game, jam out to the music and people are looking at me like I'm nuts. Where have you been? They've been paging you for an hour.

I told myself I would goof off the first week home and then get to work. I put myself on a schedule of working from 9 to 2:30 in the afternoon. Worked for a week. Finished chapter 2 of my novel.[26] Then the typewriter broke. Didn't realize how much I depend on this machine. Borrowed a manual from my friend. Something like 13 keys stuck on this thing. Got the typewriter back in a couple of weeks but by then I was on a fast downhill run. Would you believe that there is only one

---

[26]Parker did not finish her novel, but it is available in manuscript form with her papers at the Schlesinger.

typewriter repair shop that works on this brand of machine in the East Bay?

Forgive all the errors in this letter. It's been so long that I'm going to have to learn how to type all over again. That's not to say what I knew before was anything to brag about.

Gente had a retreat planned for the July 4th weekend. I almost learned how to swim. I also got very drunk and hostile. Upset a few folks. Since then I've been trying to get it together again. Been on the wagon for a little over a week. And it is difficult. So the next time you see me I'll probably [be] quiet, withdrawn, dull, but sober.

Have also got to put myself on a diet. Gained a great deal of weight. Feel like I'm dragging about triplets. Can't afford to ruin my image as a sex symbol, right?

I think someone in my neighborhood is expressing their opinion of our sexual preferences. I've had three flat tires this week. Think I'm going to have to set up in my window with a rifle or something.

Some good news – Ann is playing in a band. They call themselves "Dimly Lit." For me it's not so good. They are the rehearsingiest band in the world. However I complain not. I can adjust to having to make appointments to see my lover. At least she doesn't ask for two weeks notice.

Audre, I've got to stop this. Looking at these typing errors is driving me angry. I'll write another letter tomorrow telling you about the trip. My love to you and your family. Tell Frances[27] I've only found one bridge game since I got home. You two are going to have to come out here or all that time and learning will go for naught.

Pat

---

[27] Frances Clayton was Audre Lorde's partner for seventeen years.

July 25, 1975

Good morning love,

It's a brand new day and I feel much better. I walked out of my studio yesterday, into my bedroom and refused to leave for any reason, even Gente. Received a few phone calls inquiring about my health. I haven't missed a practice since the season started, excluding the time when I was away.

Now the trip - First let me say that your house, your family, you were the high point. When people ask me what I think of New York I tell them the only good thing in it is you and your family in Staten Island. Now I know you must disagree with my opinion, but I really didn't care for the place. I'm sure a great deal of it has to do with the women and the readings. In fact, the majority, but the situation with drivers and pedestrians really bothered me. It struck me as a great lack of respect. It also upset me when we returned to see the same thing developing here. Give us 5 years and we will be playing dodge cars too. I don't know maybe the country girl in me just can't handle the big city.

Anyway after we left your house we went to D.C. I really enjoyed our stay there. The first reading was a little strange. It was in a bar (that part isn't strange). There was a singer on the bill with me. I was not aware of this until the day of the reading. When I get to the place they start telling me about 45 minute sets. I assume 45 minutes each. They mean together. They want the singer to have more time. People relate to singers better than poets. My ego is getting uptight. I took 25 minutes the second act. The singer wasn't that damn good. The singer took an hour. Time to get paid. They want to make the split 65-35. Singers always get more than poets. My reply - "Not this poet." Got the feeling they weren't too happy with me. I got my money. Sold a lot of books. The women we stayed with in D.C. were really nice. E. Sharon Gomillion.[28] 100 pds. of energy. She set up the second reading at her house. Charged people money, provided free food and beer, sent invitations to all her friends. Incredible evening. It struck me what one of the things bothering me was. At this reading at Lois's (E. Sharon) the audience was 75% black. Oh how sweet it was. Wanted to spread my body over the entire room and touch every one of those sisters. In fact the whole city of Washington just kept me high.

In between the two readings in D.C. we went to Philadelphia. Again, I enjoyed it. Met a friend of yours. Anita.[29] She came back to Washington with us. Oh at Lois', there was this sister named Ruby. She said she had been to your house, apparently the days we went off to New Haven. I think I got you in trouble. She asked me about the tape I did with you and I said, "what type?" Listen if we are going to be doing things together that we really aren't doing together - tell me. If I could have turned red –I would have been quite red. Anyway who is this woman? I immediately took a disliking to her. Impressed me as some sort of Black groupie and a lazy one at that. Also drank up my beer with one of her dates and that didn't set right with me at all. She was crushing at Lois'. Thought at one point Lois was going to kill her. Another thing that struck me was she seemed to be trying to be a sex symbol. When she found out I had been married to Ed,[30] she decided that was why Ed had an obsession

---

[28] E. Sharon (Lois) Gomillion was a Washington, DC-based poet. Diana Press published her chapbook *Forty Acres and a Mule* in 1973.

[29] It is possible that Parker met Anita Cornwell, author of the essay collection *Black Lesbian in White America* (Naiad Press, 1983). Cornwell lived in Philadelphia.

[30] Ed Bullins was Parker's first husband. Parker and Bullins met in Los Angeles and married in June 1962; they moved to the San Francisco Bay area together, but separated and a court annulled their marriage in January 1966. Bullins was Minister of Culture for the Black Panther Party and became a noted playwright in the Black Arts Movement.

with dykes. I think it broke her heart when I told her Ed didn't know I was a dyke until '74. Strange lady.

At the party a woman from *off our backs*[31] came to do an interview.[32] And I was exhausted. When we went to Philly, they had a party after the reading and I got wasted. The next night there was the party at Lois'. I went upstairs and laid down and here comes the friendly reporter. 3 hours. And I asked her to show me the interview before it was printed in case I wanted to make changes. She comes over the next day with a page and a half of copy. I spent a great deal of time talking about the racism we had encountered both in and out of the women's community. No mention. I asked her to take out the names of the club I had read at. My comments were negative. Talking about the money incident with the singer. Then she sends me the papers and it's still there. New lesson for the kid - Beware of interviews.

We left D.C. and went to Baltimore – no reading - just to visit the women from Diana Press. Felt a strong class difference. Coletta[33] got uptight, because Ann and I went out to buy some tank tops and didn't want to go to a second hand store. And I got uptight cause I can't relate to someone telling me about working class and middle class and how much better one is than the other. After spending my first 17 years in second hand clothes have no desire to continue. I think that's one of the primary differences that turn third world women off of the women's movement. The white women are running around and talking about how bad it is to be a housewife and stay home and the third world women are trying to get there.

Then we went to Cincinnati. Small reading and people apologizing for the lack of third world women. I think before I

---

[31] A national feminist newspaper published from Washington, DC from 1970 until 2008.

[32] The interview with Parker ran in *off our backs* 4, no 4 (May-June 1975): 16.

[33] Coletta Reid, the co-owner of Diana Press.

go on tour again, I'm going to write a year in advance so those women can comb the Black communities. Some of them almost had me in tears.

Well, it is now Wednesday morning. I left the studio Friday and haven't been back since then. Went to practice Saturday, and then had to move a refrigerator. Sunday we played a game against the second place team in the League and won. Yours truly being the starting pitcher. Yea for me. Spent Monday running to the bank and moving a couch for another friend. Beginning to think that owning a truck isn't such a good idea after all. Yesterday, spent the day with Ann. She was depressed about the band. She doesn't like the music they are playing. Feeling doubtful about her abilities. Also went out to Alameda College to see about enrolling. They were closed. So, I'll go again today. I decided maybe I should go and get that piece of paper. The end of the uneducated poet.[34]

Oh throughout the weekend, when we had to go to the bars after the game, I still managed not to drink. Small pat on the back in order. Now back to the trip.

Drove to St. Louis. Scared shitless. On the radio they started issuing tornado warnings and neither Ann nor I knew what you were supposed to do in a tornado or what one looked like if we saw one. Right then I was definitely ready to come home. We stayed in St. Louis with a woman named Alma. She worked her butt off getting things set up and it showed. However, she planned this party at one of the bars for me and failed to tell me about it. We go there and here are all these people waiting to meet me and expecting me to read a little poetry, would you believe preview? The reading was the following night at Washington University. Fantastic. Really fine audience I got off and read my heart out. However the lack of third world

---

[34]Immediately after high school graduation, Parker went to Los Angeles and enrolled at Los Angeles Community College. She took college classes in the San Francisco Bay area but never completed a degree.

women still existed. There were two women there and one of them was reading on the program with me. Went back to Alma's and played bridge. Lost badly. And then there was a problem, seemed like the few people that I have run into that play the game don't know nearly as much about it as Frances. They have a hard time answering my questions. The next day we just took it easy. Went to a restaurant, ate dinner, went to a movie, and then discovered a carnival on the way home and stayed there until after midnight. Even though we had to get up at 7 am. Loved every minute of it. I get off on carnivals.

Left the next day and drove to McAlester, Oklahoma. The next day we were in Houston. So, now my problem begins of how to tell mama that her youngest child is a dyke. It took me 3 days to get up the nerve. And when I tell her all she says is, "Well, as long as you're happy it's alright with me." How anti-climactic. Here I've been building up for this moment for 8 years and that's it. Not even one tear or yell or look of shock.

Did the reading. Made sure I read all the poems about growing up in Houston and the shit I caught there. There was this Black woman from one of the Black radio stations there to do an interview. Poor child looked scared to death. She sat about three feet away from me and held the microphone out at arms length. When she realized I wasn't going to rape her or her arms got tired she moved in closer. I'm still not sure exactly what the motivation was. After the reading, they took us out to one of the local bars. The jukebox was full of country and western music and would you believe those folks got up and started square dancing. Ann and I almost busted our guts. Had the feeling we were definitely in the wrong place. And when we got up and did the bump, I thought the folks were going to faint. In fact, I had the feeling, the fact that Ann and I were together was causing a few mind problems.

In any case, Houston was fun. My mother put us to work laying down a rug for her and painting the back porch. She really enjoyed our being there. My cousin came over and barbequed for us. I blew Ann's mind a little. I had told her about being respectful to elders, and the number of relatives I had in the town, but what I forgot to tell her about was that I would have to pay visits to all the neighbors. She came back telling everybody that "And Pat knows all the neighbors on her street."

We left Houston, drove to Lordsburg, New Mexico, and the next night to L.A. Stopped off and said hello to my sisters, then came home. Never though I'd get so excited about Oakland. Well I think that covers it. If I have missed something, shoot the question back and I'll answer it.

I'm going to close up and get my butt out to Alameda. The idea of going back to school scares me. I haven't been in school for about 10 years. I worry about acquiring good study habits. I worry even more about listening to 17 and 18 year olds telling me about the world.

I'm sorry to hear about *AQ*. But don't turn your back on all such ventures. I'm in the process of trying to start a magazine out here. And I do seem to remember extracting a promise from you to handle the East Coast. That's still pretty much in the air. I'm not about the jump up or off into anything until I'm sure. And I want to make sure it's going to be something special. Ego insists on the best.

Oh, got a letter from Ann Shockley about a book of essays.[35] Wrote and told her I had read her novel. That it got me through the boredom of driving the last part of the trip. I didn't tell her that she had me in stitches. Now what exactly do you want me to do with that book? I could send it to you real fast. I could pass it on to someone else to read also.

---

[35]Ann Allen Shockley is the author of *Loving Her* (1974), *The Black and the White of It* (1980), *Say Jesus and Come to Me* (1982), and *Celebrating Hotchclaw* (2005).

Also the money you sent me when I sent *Womanslaughter*, was that from *AQ* or you and was it for the poem? If so tell me how much it was and I'll send it back.

Give my love to Frances, Jonathan and Beth.[36] Also send me Frances' last name. I'd like to write her a letter. Take care and be easy.

Oh. I'm in correspondence with a woman out here who loves you, honey. I told her I stayed at your house and she bout died. "Audre Lorde, Audre Lorde, Oh my God. Audre Lorde, the real Audre Lorde? Oh my goodness. She's just the most beautiful woman in the world. I just love her. I mean Audre Lorde!" All of the above is a verbatim quote.

Also when you write back tell me about your tomatoes. I've been picking blackberries out off my back yard. Had my first pie. Going to try to can some and if I'm successful I['ll] save some for you. Enough. This is turning into a book.

Love,
Pat

Oh, new director at Poetry Center at S. F. State. Rumor has it that he's a real pig. Not interested in Third World Poetry or Women's Poetry. Wants to bring name poets—high quality folks. Best get a letter off & tell him your name.[37]

---

[36] Jonathan Rollins-Lorde is Audre Lorde's son, born in 1964, and ten years old at the time of this letter. Beth Rollins-Lorde is Audre Lorde's daughter, born in 1963 and twelve years old at the time of this letter.

[37] This postscript is written by hand on the letter in the Spelman archive collection of Audre Lorde. The new director of the Poetry Center was Lewis MacAdams. He succeeded Kathleen Fraser and served as director for three years.

10/7 [/1975][38]

Dear Pat—

Our summer was beautiful - rock hunting in Minnesota and Lake Superior & peace & quiet. No more. The rat race has begun. And how's life with you?

This is on this paper because I sat down to compose a shit-assy letter to some shit-assy people + of course I'd rather write to you which I've been meaning to do since we returned to your pretty blue paper. (Now that was a letter that truly satisfied my soul with blow-by-blow accounts which I LOVE)

(I love knowing every little detail of what every person is doing... take heed, please.)

To answer some of your questions- Ruby is/was a troubled little sister (she's younger than she looks, who I thought I could help (when I was into the helping bag) I was wrong, altho I can't say I was defeated- she surely did give her a run for –etc. I think you hit the nail on the head- a groupie. But June Jordan and I were either too naïve or too stupid to see it. She is among other things a pathological liar. (if you didn't notice...) AS you know, *AQ* is no more.[39] Lots of pain – can't discuss. The money I once sent you and Ann had nothing to do with them. I had given a reading at a simple place in Queens when I knew I was wasting my time and when that happens it always makes me feel good to split the cash where they'd plotz if they ever knew. The enclosed is the same. If you all don't need it, pass it on to the poets or someone.

---

[38] This is a two-page handwritten letter from Lorde to Parker. The PPS originally appeared at the top of the first page; it has been moved to the end of the letter for reading convenience.

[39] *Amazon Quarterly* stopped publishing in March 1975.

I wish you two lived closer, or that the country wasn't so damn wide (sometimes). I truly miss talking, + FC[40] says you're the best bridge player she's met since she's come to NY.

Interviews suck. So does suffering.

If you're serious about the magazine, I'll do anything and everything I can to help. But I am still a little sore, please understand.

I think it's marvelous about you + college + you'll love it I think and you'll get past the garbage and Mickey Mouse. First don't let anyone put you on- learn what you want and don't be AFRAID.

Did I tell you we miss you? It was fun and I hope we can do it again. So when y'all coming back? The kids ask for you. The pictures are yum-yum: I'm getting a set and will send them to you after I get your next letter – telling me that you do want them, it shouldn't be a total waste.

10/8 They're fucking with me at work and I just might lose my job - you know of course that New York has sold itself for a mess of Beamers, and is going bankrupt. The repercussions are many and I'm trying to steer clear of them, but it's hard.[41]

Frances has gone into training at the Institute of Human Identity and is doing therapy with gay women and loves it.

I may go to Nigeria but even that's not settled yet because of the border dispatchers. Is it about FESTAC?[42]

10/9 This has gone on for three interrupted days and it's time it evolves

Audre

---

[40]Frances Clayton, Lorde's partner.

[41]Alexis De Veaux discusses tensions in the English Department of John Jay College involving the creation of a black studies program (*Warrior Poet: A Biography of Audre Lorde,* New York: W. W. Norton, 2004: 139-140).

[42]FESTAC '77 (FESTival of Art and Culture) was also called the Second World Black and African Festival of Art and Culture. It was a festival held in Lagos, Nigeria in January and February 1977.

PPS. The word sent around by L+G[43] of *AQ* is that my upset in the mag is only because I'm both paranoid + lazy (being black, y'know…) Have you heard the like? They're living right down or up the street from you.

---

[43]Laurel Galana and Gina Covina who edited and published *Amazon Quarterly*.

11 July 1977

Pat Parker
968 60th St.
Oakland, CA 94608

Dear Pat—Tried to return your call but no answer—Am back in town until 7/27. Call or write. Am still happy to do something for your new book but I must see it in order to.[44] Call me.

Love
Audre

---

[44]Lorde wrote the introduction to Parker's *Movement in Black*, published in a cloth edition by Diana Press in 1978.

August 20, 1979

Audre Lorde
207 St. Paul Avenue
Staten Island, N.Y. 10304

Dear Audre,

Pat and I crossed our wires and each thought we had written you. I'm sorry for the delay.

I would like to first thank you for your beautiful and support[ive] letter.[45] It and others like it were very important to us both personally as well as in terms of the case. The situation as it stands now is the custody for Cassidy remains in my name. We went into court prepared to establish an entire case to prove "dectroment" should Cassidy be removed from our home. We came in with psychiatrist, psychologist, family, friends, etc.... the judge, however, decided not to hear either our presentation or the natural mothers presentation but to stand by the (probation report).

In many ways this is making things difficult for us since it does establish an easy opportunity for appeal. Also, it means in the future should the mother return to court we'll have to do it all again anyway. At any rate we have Cassidy and our family is settled back into a more normal pattern. One of the most exciting parts of the situation was the probation report. The probation worker had initially been very tentative and frighten[ed] about dealing with the case. After two meetings with us however, she changed her mind and came out with a beautiful report that couldn't have been written better by us. It was very feminist, full of compassion, as well as common

---

[45]Lorde wrote a letter on behalf of Parker and Laura Brown as adoptive parents of Brett Cassidy Brown.

sense. She wrote beautiful statements regarding the positive nature of an interracial family as well as the lesbian family. We were quite excited and impress[ed] with this worker[']s courage.

Things this summer ha[ve] been slowing down since the trial. Pat has not been writing as much as she would like but is working on some new exciting projects which is keeping her going. The health center is going and doing fine we have some new women that are making things more interesting every day.

We're hoping for a visit this year and would love to have you stay with us. The house got all fixed up in a very short time to prepare for our social workers visit so now we're trying to enjoy having the house together.

Mid September, Alicia, one of the directors of the health center, and I will be in New York. I'll try and drop you a note to let you know when and give you a call when I get there.

Please say hello to your whole family. I would especially like to say that both Pat and I are concern[ed] about your mother and hope that she is well. All our good thoughts are with her.

Sincerely,
Laura[46]

---

[46]Parker and Laura Brown were intimate partners from the mid-1970s until the late 1970s.

April 29, 1980[47]

Audre Lorde
207 St. Paul Avenue
Staten Island, New York 10304

Dear Audre,

I know you must be surprised to receive a letter from me, however I am sort of cheating; I discovered these wonderful, wonderful inventions called a Dictaphone and a good typist named Denise. I hope that you and your family are well, give my love to Francis and tell her I'm still waiting for that bridge game. Now, the reason that I am writing is I have become more and more distressed each day about the political situation in this country and feeling very inadequate to respond to what I feel are some very real messages toward world war. So sitting around one night and brain storming I got this idea that perhaps there should be some type of organization for Black women but unlike any of the others that I've known. What I'm interested in is an organization that is not secular in organization, as has been in the past. It's not to be a cultural nationalist organization, it's not to be limited in its scope. I feel that now is the time for people to understand and implement coalition politics; that now is a time for an organization that addresses itself not only to the needs of Black people in this country but to have a global perspective and understand our connection with other third world countries.

I am in the process now of writing up the guidelines of goals of the organization which I have named Black Women's Revolutionary Council. I was thinking about women that I

---

[47]Parker did a draft of this letter on April 18th; she corrected then retyped and mailed the letter on April 29th.

would like to be in that organization and of course your name popped into my head, but then it occurred to me that you and I have never sat down and discussed at any great length politics, other than politics dealing with the Women's Movement and the Lesbian Movement, and this particular organization that I'm talking about goes for all Black women. I'm adding also one of the founders of another organization for women called Eleventh Hour Battalion which is open to not only Black but all women who have some of the political beliefs and understandings as the rest of the founding members and what that basically is, is that not only are we anti-sexist, racist, fascist, but also we are anti-imperialist and we are opposed to the stand that this country has taken in its dealings with other countries in the world particularly third world countries. One of our positions is that the United States should not interfere with the internal workings of any government of the world, which has gotten into some difficulty, of course, around the situation of Iran. There are many people who somehow feel that we have every right to react to the situation in Iran and take basically a "let's nuke them" position.[48]

I was thinking about doing a tour probably late Fall so there's a possibility, if you are doing one of those, rare moments at home, that I might see you, however, that's not set yet because I haven't talked to Roadwork at all to see what the feasibility of that is.[49] Soon as I have some more information about that I will drop a line or call and let you know what's happening there.

---

[48] Parker gave the speech, "Revolution: It's Not Neat or Pretty or Quick" at the BASTA conference in Oakland, California in August 1980; a fair transcription of the speech was included in *This Bridge Called My Back* (Watertown, MA: Persephone Press, 1981; Kitchen Table Woman of Color Press, 1983: 238-242). The essay is included in *The Complete Works of Pat Parker* (254-9).

[49] Roadwork was a national multi-racial, cross-cultural women's arts organization based in Washington, DC.

We ran into Felicia about a month, month and a ½ ago and she seemed to be pretty much ok, I talked to her about a hour; suggested that she get in touch with you because I felt like you would probably be interested in hearing from her and knowing how she was. She said that she would do that, but then you know Felicia, so if you've gotten a letter, yeah she did it and if you haven't, well, par for the course.

I just flashed on one of the things I would like for the Black Women's Revolutionary Council to get into is simply dispensing of information. I went to lunch today in a Black restaurant here in Oakland and as I was sitting at the table I noticed that they were serving Hunt's Catsup. The thought struck me that probably the owners of that restaurant had no idea about H. L. Hunt and how he spends his money trying to undermine the position of Black people in this country and that it would be a very simple thing to gather that kind of information and pass it on to Black radio stations, newspapers, and simply to make up flyers, basically form letters to people like that restaurant owner so that they don't in fact spend their money and give it to organizations that are working against their interest. Those are some of the things I figure people can do, who were still not in a position to take a much more militant, revolutionary stand- understandably that's not an easy position for one to come to. Unfortunately the thing I'm worried about is that this government may not give us any chance at all to form any kind of grass roots organization. We may all find ourselves in war within the next 2 or 3 months. In fact it might not even be 2 or 3 months. I just listened to part of Jimmy Carter's speech today about Iran and to be perfectly frank it scares the shit out of me.[50]

---

[50] On April 24, 1980, President Jimmy Carter ordered Operation Eagle Claw to attempt to end the hostage crisis and rescue the fifty-two embassy staff people held in Iran. The operation failed and the hostage crisis—and tensions between the United States and Iran—heightened.

I read the article that you wrote in *Conditions* 5[51] and smiled a lot; inwardly it made me feel very good. It was definitely something that was necessary and should have been written, and I think the thing that I was most impressed by were the people that you had around. It made me feel real good knowing that you had people around you who are loving and caring and could do that in a way that gave you strength. I think that's something that we probably all need, but then you know that. I mean that's probably what you were trying to tell me way back long time ago in that apartment on Cole Street. As to more familial things, both Laura and Cassidy are fine; we've been in court one time since the last time I talked to you and the outcome of that basically was that there was no visit from the natural mother at Christmas and there was a visit scheduled for Easter but that one didn't come off. The woman decided that they didn't really have the money and couldn't afford it. Apparently her old man works for Chrysler Corporation and at some point he was laid off. The situation in the probation department is somewhat tenuous at this point. Proposition 9, which is very similar to the Briggs amendment, but is specifically directed to the State Government and its spending of funds is threatening to put an end to places like the probation department; so things are a little shaky except the latest polls are indicating that maybe Prop 9 won't pass.[52] I think people are beginning to realize that all of the good that Prop 13 theoretically was going to do in reality hit them in places that they don't like to be hit, less police departments, less fire departments, less extra curriculum activities at schools;

---

[51]Lorde's piece "Tar Beach" appeared in *Conditions Five: The Black Women's Issue* (Autumn 1979): 34-47.

[52]The Briggs Amendment, also known as the Briggs Initiative and California Proposition 6, was a ballot question on the November 1978 ballot that would have prevented gay men and lesbians—and possibly anyone who supported gay rights—from working in the California Public Schools; the proposition was defeated at the polls. In June 1980, California voters considered Proposition 9, a constitutional amendment on taxes; this proposition failed as well.

things that people get a little nervous and uptight about.[53] The status right now in the case is, well it's really difficult to say, the original judge just moved to another department, the new judge is a very young, white, liberal. Seems like somebody that would hear our case and wouldn't automatically go besonkers, because we're lesbians. The attorney thinks that we're in a really good position, particularly considering the lack of attention by the natural mother; not doing the two visits, not calling on her birthday, not calling on Christmas, just general shabby, "I don't really give a damn about this kid, but I'm just going to fight you because I don't want you dykes to have her" attitude. The next scheduled visit would be some time this summer and so we will have to wait and see if that happens, what happens etc. All in all, things here have been basically good. The one thing I have not been doing for quite a long time is writing, which is beginning to turn me into some what of a grouch and a bitch. I am trying to order things in my life so that within the next couple of months I can devote myself to writing almost exclusively. I've had some good ideas that I'd like to get a chance to work at and see what happens around.

I'm assuming that things with your family are well; that you and your daughter have come to some type of understanding that is mutually acceptable by both of you - also assuming that the situation with your mother is in good shape. I make these assumptions based on that if the shit was really bad that somehow you would call me or contact me or word would get to me. I am still a strong believer that the lesbian grapevine has got to be one of the most thorough means of communication known to mankind and just wish I could figure out a way, how we could implement and use that device for a lot better things than gossip.

---

[53]California voters passed Proposition 13 in June 1978; the proposition limited state property tax.

I feel somewhat hampered trying to communicate by writing a letter. I look forward to the time when you and I can sit down for a very long period of time and talk out a lot of the things that have been happening to us and happening between us. I think, in fact I know, there have been some misunderstandings on both our parts and would really like things to be cleared up. I do value very much you as a person and your friendship and would hate to see that deteriorate. Again, I hope that all things are well in your life and the goddess is being good to you; so until I either see you, call you, or write a letter again, take care.

With love,
Pat

[June 1980][54]

Dear Pat – I'd like to present 10-15 minutes of your work, along with other "L" women "poets," at the International Festival of Women Artists in Copenhagen. If there's any problem with this or if you have a special preference for what's read, please contact me before July 13th, I'll be back in August.

    Love,
    Audre

---

[54]This letter was on a small note card with Lorde's Staten Island address on it and sent to Parker on 12th Avenue in Oakland, California.

2/16/83

Dear Pat – It was good to see you again. I'm sorry we did not have more time to talk!

The enclosed check is part of what I feel belongs to you as a sister Poet from what I was paid in Europe, given that you did one reading + I did two. It would be more but I also paid for Barbara's transportation.[55]

I think the financial matters in Europe were handled very badly, altho I'd like to believe it was bad planning rather than any one person being to blame. So this is the only way I can see to try and make sense out of it all.

I feel it is very important, Pat, for you and I to maintain some kind of clarity between us about such matters, financial + otherwise, since I have the feeling that this is not the only time we have been used against each other in petty ways.

I hope your plans for the baby work out, and that they bring you much joy.[56]

In the hand of Afrekete,[57]

Love
Audre

---

[55]Parker and Lorde read together in October 1983 at the University of Oregon. De Veaux writes: "While Lorde thought no one person was to blame, she felt that the financial arrangements were badly handled, wanted to be sure things between herself and Parker were clear, and was concerned the money matter might be used to pit them against each other in some petty ways" (*Warrior Poet*, 168). It is possible that the Barbara to whom Lorde refers is Barbara Smith.

[56]Parker and her partner Martha Dunham were in the process of adopting a child together.

[57]Afrekete is the symbolic black lesbian that Lorde identifies in *Zami: A New Spelling of My Name*.

[Spring 1985][58]

Dear Pat

Happy Spring to you + your family. Please come out from behind your computer long enough to say hello! I'm looking forward so much to your new book, and haven't heard from you in a while about your coming out this way. I won't bore you with why I've disappeared, but with the exception of June when Francis + I will be in Vermont and 8/15-9/15 when I'll be in Australia I'll be here, and we would both love to have you stay in lovely scenic downtown Staten Island! And Marty, of course. I could even hang for Redtop and the better one, too! So let me know, Old Girl, and don't make me feel like I'm chasing after you again.

Life gets stranger and stranger in a good or heavy way. So far, the second baby has not been less beautiful - I'd been sort of happy for some rest I think. A lot's been taking off with Art Against Apartheid and SISA, which Gloria Joseph + I are literally dragging into existence. Sisters in Support of Sisters in South Africa.[59]

Francis is well and the kids are big and beautiful. Beth graduates in June. Jonathan's got another year to go & a live in lady at Vassar. I went to Cuba in January-quite a trip! Write me.

I love you.
Audre

---

[58]This letter is dated based on Lorde's travel using De Veaux's biography, *Warrior Poet*.

[59]SISA is the acronym for Sisterhood in Support of Sisters in South Africa.

November 13, 1985

Dear Audre,

I do hope you are sitting so the shock doesn't boil you over. I received a request from Frances Phillips to read with you in February at the Women's Building.[60] I am always pleased to read with you and I look forward to seeing you. This letter is an informal formal invitation to you to come and stay with me and my family while you are in the area. If you don't give me too hard a time when you come, I'll even let you loose on my word processor.

I was disappointed that I wasn't able to see you while I was in New York, but I felt your vibes, honey. Did Frances go with you? I called her several times and never got an answer, so I thought maybe she decided to hit the road with you for a change.

The tour was probably one of the best things that could have happened to me. I had returned from Europe feeling really down and egoless. I saw a copy of Judy Grahn's book and discovered I wasn't a lesbian poet. That hurt.[61] I still haven't been able to resolve how I'm going to deal with Judy from this point. I really don't understand what that was about. It's so contradictory to everything we've talked about and done in the past in regards to competition and divisiveness among women poets. In any case, I was feeling low.

Hitting the road turned that around for me. I was very pleasantly surprised by the response of audiences everywhere I went. I was ready to pack up and move to Boston and

---

[60]The Women's Building in San Francisco, founded in 1971, is a community space that hosts many cultural and arts events.

[61]Parker refers to Judy Grahn's *The Highest Apple,* a collection of essays about lesbian poets.

Manhattan. (That is a joke.) It did make me realize that there are still people out there who believe in me and my work.

So then I got angry. I decided that the way to prevent people from dismissing me and what I'm doing is to do so much more of it that it's impossible for them to get away with it.

Obviously I didn't reach this great insight right away. I took all sorts of other diversions. I started some seriously heavy drinking, hanging out in bars and had an affair. I managed to come out of this with my relationship with Marty still intact, bruised like hell, but intact.

Started seeing a therapist with Marty and individually and it's proved to be quite helpful despite my resistance. It's hard for us strong Black women types to admit we're fucking falling apart at the seams as you must well know. Out of all this madness, and I really do believe I was mad, I've come to some decisions that are as scary as hell, but at the same time are exciting.

I informed the women at the Health Center that I am leaving effective January 1st.[62] I am going to come home to my machine and do what I've always wanted. Write. I've talked this over and over with Marty and she is being absolutely wonderful and supportive. She's helping me compile a mailing list to try and get readings to supplement my income and we've worked out a budget and looked at where we can cut back and cut out and off to make it, so that the pressure of earning money isn't so great that I have to spend all my time hustling gigs and still not get the writing done.

I'm reading everything I can find in the library about starting a small business and taxes, and agents and markets. I would be really appreciative if you could tell me everything you think I

---

[62]Parker worked as an administrator at the Oakland Feminist Women's Health Center.

need to know around any of these issues and if you think of something I haven't mentioned, please tell me.

It means I'll have to give up things like my weekly lobster or crab and I definitely can't afford to hang out in the bars and drink, but it also means I get to take that shot. I've never had the opportunity to write full time and that has me jumping up and down.

Given how fast I usually work when I write, I don't see any reason why I can't do a novel in a year as well as a book of poems. It means I finally get to see how good I really am or how bad.

Right now, I'm so pumped up from the excitement that my confidence is soaring, but still have the other voice that says "what if?" Working full time at the Health Center has always been a built-in excuse for not producing. If I fall on my face, I'm not real sure how I'll handle it. Promoting myself has never been one of my strong points, and I know I'll have to do a certain amount of it to make this work. I can't be dependent on Marty for too long.

I know you know, but I'll say it anyway. I'm going to need your help.

Pat

December 6, 1985

Dear Pat,

I sit in this place to write you, wanting to do it in my own hand but wanting also the clear precisions of this machine that becomes like an excising filter, sharp, inexorable. I love the way colored girls always get the message—your call, after this letter was framed and ready to jump out my eyes onto some page. Between its intent and conception after receiving yours, and the present now, has been, as I told you, difficult days for me. But I am strong and feisty and fighting all the way. Did a benefit reading with Cheryl Clarke for a new lesbian magazine the students at Hunter are starting for the University as a whole and it gave me an enormous charge to feel what such an event could mean just in terms of change and the world's story and us, etc. and looking at their wonderful young faces?[63] I felt very blessed to be who I am and where I was and a part of it all.

I have always loved you, Pat, and wanted for you those things you wanted deeply for yourself. Do not think me presumptuous—from the first time I met you in 1970 I knew that included your writing. I applaud your decision. I support you with my whole heart and extend myself to you in whatever way I can make this more possible for you. I hope you know by now I call your name whenever I can and will continue to do so. But you're right, you don't want to tie yourself up with so many gigs you don't have good solid time to stare at the walls and read the words stitched into the cracks between the nail holes.

Frances was still in Vermont when you were here and I was in NZ. She may be visiting too when I come up to SF in February, in which case we'll want a nice sound-proofed room

---

[63]*The Olivetree Review* started in 1982 and continues to publish today.

with a big bed. Otherwise I will be real pleased to stay with you and Marty—I've been wanting to feel you and your family.

When I did not receive an answer to my letter last spring, I took a long and painful look at the 15 years we have known each other and decided that I had to accept the fact that we would never have the openness of friendship I always thought could be possible being the two strong Black women we are, with all our differences and samenesses. Then your card from Nairobi,[64] and I thought once again maybe when I'm out there next spring Pat and I will sit down once and for all and look at why we were not more available to each other all these years. I was overjoyed to get your letter and what it means in your life. There are conversations we need to have, Pat, each for her own clarity, and neither one of us has forever.

over

Things you must beware of right now---

A year seems like a lot of time now at this end—it isn't. It took me three years to reclaim my full flow. Don't lose your sense of urgency on the one hand, on the other, don't be too hard on yourself—or expect too much.

Beware the terror of not producing

Beware the urge to justify your decision.

Watch out for the kitchen sink and the plumbing and that painting that always needed being done. But remember the body needs to create too.

Beware feeling you're not good enough to deserve it

Beware feeling you're too good to need it

Beware all the hatred you've stored up inside you, and the locks on your tender places.

Frances and I leave for Switzerland 12/14. If you write to me the address is

---

[64]Parker went to Nairobi in 1985 as a part of women's delegation to raise awareness about domestic violence; she read her poem "Womanslaughter."

Prof. Audre Lorde
Lukas Klinik
CH-4144 Arlesheim
SWITZERLAND

I'll be there certainly until the 7th, probably until the 12th. I'd love to hear from you, and we will talk then. May this coming new year be a rich and fruitful one for you, Pat, and for those you love.

In the hand of Afrekete,
Love,
Audre

February 16, 1986

Audre,

I wanted to get this letter off to you while you and my thoughts are still fresh in my mind. Too often in the past, I have put letter writing off, because I thought whatever free time I had had to go to those survival things and if any energy left over would go to writing. However, it does occur to me that letter writing is both a survival thing and writing, plus it is so important to me to continue our conversation.

I can't ever remember having enjoyed the presence of anyone so much in my home. You really are a bright light and are perhaps the best person in the world for shaking me out of my propensity for laziness and self-pity. Do you think there's anyway to bottle you so one can simply ingest you when necessary, or is there any way to speed up your move to the West.

I made an assumption here that your move will be to Northern California. You wouldn't move to Los Angeles or heaven forbid San Diego? AH!!!

Marty was totally impressed with you. She hadn't mentioned it to me before your arrival, but she was a little scared. Somehow, I had never mentioned to her that Frances was white and she was afraid you would be disapproving of either her or our relationship because she is white. So when she walked into the house and was greeted by your radiant pearly whites she was totally won over.

In the past we have had quite a bit of "black nationalist" rhetoric flowing through here. I was very glad to hear your last poem, and where the hell is my copy?

I went out and found Luisah Teish's book.[65] Absolutely delightful. Also took your advice and promptly send off for a subscription to "Coda."[66] It's obvious to me that I have to turn over a certain amount of money during this year or I will mind fuck myself to death. So, obviously, I am extremely grateful to you for including me in your reading. You can't imagine how good it felt to give Marty money the night after the reading. I know on one hand that the demand is not there from Marty, but I am such a proud bitch and so used to paying my own way. I also know if I can contribute to this household in some way no matter how small, it will help thwart off some of that self-doubt that us strong Black amazons supposedly don't have, but as we know sits on the right shoulder constantly talking shit.

Girlfriend, your departure from this state was right on time. We have been hit by a storm that is unbelievable. Had it happened while you were here, we could have taken a row boat to our reading. Flash floods, mud slides, people being evacuated from their homes, power outages for hours and in some cases days, because the repair crews can't get in to fix the lines. Intense!

We had to bring the dogs in for fear of them being washed away.

I'm going to enclose a copy of your poem with this letter.[67] Know that it will probably change, and when it does, I'll send you the revisions. Please don't be too embarrassed, it really was done out of love.

---

[65] Luisah Teish's book *Jambalaya: The Natural Woman's Book of Personal Charms and Natural Rituals* originally published in 1985.

[66] *Coda: Poets & Writers Newsletter* was published by Poets & Writers, Inc., in New York. In September/October 1980, the newsletter featured articles on women's publishing.

[67] Parker included a draft of her poem "For Audre" in the letter.

Going to close this up. Please take care of yourself and give my love to Frances. I look forward to seeing her.

Love,
Pat

P.S. How do you cook beets?

June 8, 1986

Audre,

I decided that your reply to my letter in February must be lost in the mail someplace, so I figured I'll go ahead and write you anyhow.

I got my VCR fixed, so I'm sending along your copy of "Go Tell It On The Mountain."[68] Enjoy.

Things here have been hectic as usual. Trying to get order in one's life is a trip after years of chaos. I've just returned from the Midwest. Did a speech in Columbus for a "Take Back the Night" rally and then a reading in Bloomington at the National Women's Music Festival. They both went well. The conference in Bloomington was attended by a number of producers of women's concerts, etc. Hopefully, I prove to them that there is a place for poetry at these types of functions. It still amazes me that I have to still be out here proving and reproving all the damn time.

While I was at the conference, I did a poetry-writing workshop with a bunch of little people. Great fun. I'd forgotten, how much I enjoyed working with kids in schools. I also met with Susie Gaines, booking agent for Kate Clinton, who painted a pretty dismal picture of the chances of making any money reading for universities.[69]

Returned home and have been giving myself a serious talking to about my future. Had allowed myself quite a few diversions. Starting playing softball, which in itself was alright, but following practicing and games, I found myself going to the bar and hanging out. So, this week, I went on the wagon, and have been running like a bandit from any booze.

---

[68] A film adaptation directed by Stan Lathan of Baldwin's book *Go Tell It On the Mountain* from 1984 aired; Parker recorded it on a VCR.

[69] Kate Clinton is a lesbian stand-up comedian who toured widely.

The next goal is to make myself write every day, if only for an hour. And for me this is seriously difficult. Wonder why I didn't decide to be a singer or something. The loneliness of writing drives me nuts sometimes. Notice when it's going bad, it's loneliness and when it's going good it's solitude.

Planted seeds for a garden. I have corn (two types), broccoli, peas, squash, cabbage, collards, spinach, chard, lettuce, tomatoes, and watermelon growing in egg cartons on the patio. I've already put some tomatoes, squash, and bell pepper in the ground. So, on your next trip out, my love, I'll feed you fresh, organic vegetables.

I have to close this up, I've got a meeting at the Health Center in 15 minutes. This means I'm already late. Please answer this one, or I promise to keep writing and will purposefully make each succeeding letter more boring than the last.

Give my love to Frances. When are you coming out? (as in moving?) How is your health? How is Frances's health? Did you intend to leave "This Book is Not For You" here?

Marty is doing well. She's also playing softball. She got hit in the eye at the second practice and it almost ended her career as a jock before it got started, but she is healed and well.

Stasia from time to time asks where are you? Trying to explain distance and different States to a three year old is a trip. I think she believes you are still flying around on an airplane.

I really do have to stop this. Take care.

Love,
Pat

[June or July 1986][70]

Dear Pat,

Of course this is the story of my life--, I settle down to write you a long newsy letter filled with all the things I've been meaning to send you and spend the next hour looking for the snapshots I can't find any longer in the weltering madness that is the photo box! I found one set though, so here are some of Anastasia and you and Ad.,[71] but I had some great ones of you and you and me so when I happen upon them at 3am some morning I promise I'll put them in a time capsule and shoot them off to you and Marty, who is in one great action shot.

So, girl, how's it hanging? I love your letters, when you get off your kiester and write them, and it's a damn sight easier for you because you have that magic machine that smiles and winks. I on the other hand sit here in front of this typewriter at 6am trying to talk to my friend. Who won't be up for another six hours so I can't even give up the ghost and telephone. Patti, I'm really good. The time in Europe was wonderful—affirming and invigorating—those Afro-European women are coming on, do you hear me? The sisters are coming on. It makes me feel like I've been doing good work since I was there in '84. And besides, Amsterdam is a really swinging city. You should make it your business to go—you are known and read over there, Pat, and you need to see what a difference your work has made in Black Lesbians lives on an international level. Talk to Nancy B. about Ann Dekker, who used to be with SARA Feminist Pub in Holland,

---

[70]This time estimate is based on De Veaux's chronology in *Warrior Poet* (Jonathan enrolled at Vassar in August 1982).

[71]Anastasia is the daughter of Parker and Martha Dunham; Ad. is Adrienne Rich.

and now has a press of her own.[72] Anyway, that's how I think at 6 am in the morning.

Health wise I'm hanging in, gained 10 pounds which makes me feel really good (I was not born to be insubstantial and that's how I was feeling last Feb when I saw you). Jonathan graduated from Vassar in May and Beth is the light in a lot of people's lives. Frances has forgiven me for spending the last 7 months out of NY now she's seen my test results and the scales, and we are going off to Gualala for a real vacation in August, please, no earthquakes.[73] I will call you when we're there.

That was so splendid of you to make that tape of Baldwin's and send it, I didn't think you'd remember. And you did, and we both thank you. (It's a good repro, too!)

I carry Stas' pictures around in my brag book and say, "See, here's Pat's daughter," and they're all suitably impressed, and should be. She's really a special kid.

One of the things transcendent was a chance to sit down with a group of South African women in the south of France for a week—the Zamani Soweto Sisters—a sewing collective SISA helps support. It was a wonderful sharing of strengths and pain and singing and dancing and fury and laughter and a quite extraordinary time. I draw upon it in my fury at what that Washington pig is doing in our name, aiding and abetting the Botha regime.[74] Oh, Patti! Where will we all be on Coronation Day?[75]

---

[72]Nancy B. is Nancy Bereano, the publisher of Firebrand Books. An Dekker ran a socialist feminist publishing company, SARA, in the Netherlands during the 1990s with her partner, poet Ankie Peypers.

[73]A small town in Mendocino County, California.

[74]P. W. Botha was the leader of South Africa from 1978 until 1989.

[75]Coronation Day is the celebration of the British monarchy.

Give my love to Marty and the baby, and I'll send those snaps when I find them, and call me when we get out of the hot-tub in Gualala.

Love,
Audre

August 1, 1986

Dear Audre,

Smiles and winks! This machine doesn't smile and wink. It torments me. Says so you want to be a writer huh? And presents me with a life time of blank pages. Ah!! Why didn't I want to be a carpenter, or pilot or president?

Your ears must have been burning love, cause you were definitely on my brain. I went out to Ollies a week or two ago and who walks through the door but Andrea Canaan and her lover.[76] She was coming here visiting and the letter she sent to me saying she was coming came back to her house.[77]

She was planning to go out to the tree where Jacquelyn Peters was found and leave flowers. Are we ready for lynchings in Contra Costa county?[78] Somehow I deluded myself in believing that I had seen my last body hanging from a tree when I left Texas.[79]

Sister love, the shit is scaring me. The fascists are getting bolder and bolder and the people are eating up this patriotic, nationalistic madness. I listen to the call in radio shows and it makes me want to go out and buy a machine gun. Folks are

---

[76] Andrea Canaan is a writer; her work was included in *This Bridge Called My Back*.

[77] This sentence is an awkward construction; Canaan sent a letter to Parker informing her of her visit, but the letter did not reach Parker and was instead returned to Canaan.

[78] Contra Costa County is the county in the northern part of the East Bay in the San Francisco-Oakland area of California. On November 2, 1985, Timothy Lee, a 23-year-old Black gay man, was hung to death in Concord. For more information see the footnote on page 468 of *The Complete Poems of Pat Parker*. In late June 1986, Jacquelyn Peters, a thirty-five year old black woman from Concord, California, was found hanging from an olive tree in a bank parking lot in Lafayette. Her death was initially deemed "suspicious" and then later ruled a suicide.

[79] Parker addresses lynching in her poem "Timothy Lee."

losing their minds. You would think that the lessons of the 30's and 40's would be enough, but either people's' memories are short or their knowledge of history is limited, but compared to the madness that I think is coming, Hitler was a choir boy. We are not going to have to deal with one maniac, but a whole nation of maniacs.

Gualala? You know little colored children who are educated in segregated school systems learn little about geography, especially about places where other colored folks live. So, I went to my "Hammond's World Atlas" and found no Gualala. Then I went to my dictionary: Webster's New Twentieth Century Unabridged Second Edition. I found no Gualala. Now, this is distressing, because that means you are somewhere off in the world and I can't visualize where.

Amsterdam, huh. I think I'll run right out there and get myself a ticket. Seriously, I would love to go there, but unless the salaries for unemployed poets make a sudden and drastic leap, it's not going to be possible. Although one of my ex-lovers who lives in Italy has offered to pay my way to Europe and with a Euro rail pass one could conceivably make their way there, I'd have to face the real possibility of divorce if I took her up on that offer. Maybe divorce and death.

I'm glad to hear your health is hanging and your weight improving. "Insubstantial?" Try flat out skinny, child. I was seriously getting ready to break out the chitterlings and hog maws.

The last two weeks here have been horrendous. Major problems at the Health Center and of course yours truly gets phone calls when that happens. So I've been working approximately 10 hours a day for the last 14 days, but the crisis is pretty much over and I'm back in my studio. I get so torn between here and the Center. But I can't let the last eight years of my life go for nothing. That place is too important to me. And right now it is on such shaky ground.

I'm gearing up to go after the NEA again.[80] If you have any suggestions as to how I can pull this off, please let me know. These people and their consistent rejection are beginning to piss me off.

I just finished doing an article for "Hotwire" magazine.[81] That's a first. Prose is a trip and a half. It's really weird to think in terms of expanding words and thoughts instead of honing everything down to gleaming.

Going to close this up. I'm glad you wrote and sent the pictures. I still need to develop the ones I have along with the other ten rolls that are sitting up on the counter.

I'm pleased to hear that your family is doing well, but the thought of Jonathan graduating from college makes me feel absolutely ancient however I expect those thoughts will subside when Anastasia Jean hits the door this evening. She makes me feel young and tired.

Kiss Frances for me and give her my love. I'll talk to you when you return from the place I can't see.

Love,
Pat

---

[80]The National Endowment for the Arts offers fellowships to writers and translators to support individual creative work. The NEA never awarded Parker a fellowship. For an analysis of the NEA and lesbian writers see Julie R. Enszer, "'She Who Shouts, Gets Heard!': Counting Women Writers in NEA Grants and Norton Anthologies," *Feminist Studies*, vol. 42, no. 3: 720-737.

[81]Parker's piece, "Poetry at Women's Music Festivals: Oil and Water," appeared in *Hot Wire* in 1986. It is reproduced in *The Complete Works of Pat Parker*.

January 04, 1988

Dear Sister Love,

I have no idea where to begin this letter. There are so many thoughts, and fears, and emotions moving within me that I feel like a nuclear reactor out of control. So, I am going to apologize up front for the tone and content of this letter; not for what I'm about to say, but simply because in a lot of ways hearing this must be somewhat like being in a relationship with someone a lot younger than yourself. One can find oneself retracing a lot of familiar ground.

It has taken me a long time to come to this machine. I have been avoiding this room and I'm not totally sure why. I do have some definite ideas. Today, I put a new diskette into the machine which is just for you. How's that for optimism? I'm already frustrated, because of typing errors. What little skill I possessed has eroded to the point of non-existence. Be thankful, honey chile that this is a computer or you wouldn't be able to read this. I told myself coming in here this morning that I would finish this letter no matter what. I have an unfinished letter on another disk that I started to you when I returned from the March on Washington.[82] If I add that letter to all the letters I write to you in my bed you'd be inundated with missiles for here, but we both know that what's written in your head can't be read.

I brought you up to date on the medical stuff so far on the phone.[83] Today I go to what is hopefully my last visit to the surgeon. But then as I think about it probably not. I'm beginning to think I shouldn't predict shit, because I've been

---

[82]Parker wrote an article about the 1987 March on Washington for *Hot Wire;* it is included in *The Complete Works of Pat Parker*.

[83]Parker was being treated for breast cancer.

so wrong so much of the time lately. The key word in the preceding sentence is "hopefully."

I've gotten back most of the mobility in my arm and shoulder. I must admit that I freaked out when I realized that the motion was happening. The surgeon had told me to exercise the arm and I did, but around day four post-surgery, I couldn't stand to move it. Talk about pain. Almost shocked me white. So, of course I did what was so natural and stop moving the arm altogether. Assumed what I now call the claw position. So of course the next time I see the surgeon, he's going "hey you gotta move." Now I am probably the world's worst when it comes to exercise. Like okay bore me to death. So I handled the problem my way. You want Parker to move, put a ball in the vicinity. So following my physician's advice to take more pain medication and move that arm, I returned to my gym and took more pain medication and played racquetball. I lost all three games, but I got the arm moving. Now I can unlock my top lock. Could probably comb my hair, but my sister came up from L.A. and corn rowed it, so there's no need. Still can't move it straight up over my head, but I'm working on it.

During our conversation, you mention that "adenocarcinoma" was good, as in better than some other possibilities. Why? I've not come across breaking down the types of cancer and pros and cons or if I did I was still too much in shock for it to take hold. It occurs to me that I may have to go and reread about five or six books that I read right after the biopsy. So please let me know what you've read about this.

I've decided to go with chemotherapy. As I say this, my body recoils from the screech, blow, moan, disgust, disappointments that I'm projecting to you. Hold it, Lorde. Do not send me back one of your nasty how dare you letters. I already know it is totally unfair and undeserved for me to be projecting anything to you. You have been one of the few people who have not tried to tell me what to do or perhaps in the case of chemo I should say tried to tell me what "not" to do. I have grown weary from the "help and concern" of my friends. My ex-lover's mother, who is also the grandmother of Cassidy and acts as grandmother to Anastasia is getting on every nerve I have. She's not being overly pushy, but she has let me know that she thinks any kind of "invasive" techniques i.e. biopsy, mastectomy, chemo are not only dangerous, but in fact is a form of suicide. She feels that my chances of survival are better if I do nothing. Nothing does include dietary changes. I'm not trying to present this woman's case as if she's an idiot. Her theory is not a bad one, but it's not the one for me and she does not see that to continue to present her case at this point is to be of no help at all. I do not need to go into this madness with a chorus of "you're killing yourself" ringing in my ears.

It seems to me that I understand any of the materials that I have been reading that the most crucial element in this entire process is my mind. That if I do not believe in whatever treatment I'm doing then I will not survive it. Perhaps this is too simplistic, but it's the core to me. And I am just too chicken shit to trust diet and visualization alone to effect a cure. I am also too chicken shit to trust chemo alone too. And of course the frustrating thing about all of this madness is that one will never know for sure. If I live five years from now, both sides can claim a victory of sorts. And if I die, then both can blame the other for my demise. Or more likely, I'll be blamed.

I've spent a great amount of time trying to figure out the why's of this and I keep coming out angry. All this time, I have been thinking that I have survived this system, have managed to place in a controllable state and I see this disease as a clear message that I have failed. I'm sure that I let too much of the anger turn inward and yet, I cannot see how I could have done otherwise. I tried to write it manageable, to play sports it manageable, to drink it manageable, to love it manageable. I cannot see what else I could have done here. Unless it was to do all of the above more (except drink). I would love to see what James Baldwin has to say about this shit.

Now, you realize that I am getting myself more frustrated. If I fully accept my theory that anger is the primary cause of my having cancer then I must look around me and make assessment. Why am I angry? Who am I angry at? And what can I do to change it? And of course, the minute I start thinking along this vein, I get even more angry. From the monumental thought of overthrowing the system and ridding my life of capitalism, racism, sexism, classism, to the smallest nuisance of getting Marty to put the toilet paper on the spool with the sheets unfolding outward, there is simply too much for me to handle. Ah ha, fool she says, didn't I tell you to build up support and learn to depend on people.

Sister love, sister love, sister love. We are not talking anything simple or easy here. I have been trying and getting so frustrated here. From the moment Marty talked to you on the phone and you said to call everybody you know [to ask for help], the child has been busy. This week, and it has been almost a month since my mastectomy, is the first time I have had any real time alone. She has set up a schedule of people to keep me company and make sure I don't get depressed, and these folks are getting me depressed and driving me fucking nuts. First, there are the folks who look at me like I have one foot in the grave. I fully expect them to ask me what kind of frigging casket I want, and, Audre, they whisper when they talk to me. Is cancer supposed to make my hearing super sensitive or what? Then I get the inquisitive ones who feel I must now be the local breast cancer authority and feel perfectly free to ask me everything they wanted to know about breast cancer. And then I get the person who thinks I'm totally helpless and wants to help me piss. And none of them act like it's okay for me to just sit and not talk. It's like [if] I just sit silent, then I must be depressed.

So, I finally asked Marty, probably begged is more like it, to please give me a break from so much help. Just to have people come on the days when I need to go to the doctor or someplace and then only for the time that I need to do that and this only until I can drive again which I'm hoping the surgeon will free me up to do today. Laura has agreed to trade cars with me; she has a car with power steering and automatic transmission.[84]

Now, I don't want to sound ungrateful. I really do appreciate the people who have come out for me, but I don't think I'm quite ready. And realize that some things I definitely need to work on. I noticed that I was extremely reluctant in fact would not allow anyone to help me bathe or shower except Marty. Somehow it just didn't seem right or comfortable and I know I need to change that. Of course, this realization comes with my ability to do it myself, but it is difficult for me to ask for help if I think there's a remote chance that I can do it myself.

Anastasia seems to be handling this well. We managed to sneak her into the hospital and at first she was afraid, because Marty had explained that the hospital staff might make her leave, but once she figured out they were not going to, then she fell into a normal mode. She has seen the surgery scars and touched all the pertinent places. She seems more concerned about the fact that my "stomach is big" in the absence of the breast. From time to time she forgot that jumping on me hurt, but she's basically got it figured out now. I think at one point, she was somewhat jealous of the attention that I was getting from Marty, but since then she has decided to help Marty take care of me. For Christmas, I bought her a car. Yes, a real life, put your feet on the pedal and go car. It has a battery that is rechargeable and goes up to two and a half miles per hour in forward and reverse. First thing she wanted to know was if she could drive herself to school. As soon as we get some photos

---

[84]Laura Brown, Parker's ex-lover and co-parent to Cassidy.

developed, I'll send them along. Speaking of photos, did I send you the photos that we took in the front yard with Adrienne?

Last week I went to the gym. Had a good time playing racquetball, but totally freaked out about any of the other woman there seeing me minus Myrtle. Myrtle Schwartz was a fictitious person we invented at the Health Center and who people (bill collectors) were referred to until we could figure out a way to pay them in the old days. So, the gone breast immediately became Myrtle in my mind. My reaction surprised me since I didn't think I had any unusual attachments to any part of my body except my eyes. I was afraid to go into the locker room and undress alone. I waited until Marty had changed and then had her come over and help me. And in reality I think I could have undressed myself without help, but I needed to have Marty there for support. I have not been able to walk around that locker room without a towel over my scar. So why all the apprehension of a group of folks that I don't even know? In fact, since the surgery, I have not been to the gym without Marty, and that's totally different from the old days.

I've got to close this up. I'm due at the surgeon's, but I do have one more question? In your book, you mentioned Andrea Canaan and a look she gave you.[85] I just got a letter from her saying she is going to be out here at the end of the month and wants to come and stay here overnight. Good idea? Bad idea?

I've also decided that I still have a great deal more to say so instead of closing this and getting it in the mail before the doctor's visit, I am going to put this in memory and finish it when I return home and mail it tomorrow.

---

[85]In *A Burst of Light,* which Parker was probably reading in manuscript or galleys (the book was published in May 1988), Lorde writes of Andrea Canaan, "I spoke with Andrea in New Orleans this morning. She and Diana are helping to organize a Black Women's Book Fair. Despite its size, there is not one feminist bookstore in the whole city. She's very excited about the project, and it was a real charge talking to her about it" (100).

Well, we've returned from the doctor's appointment and I was right to think that maybe I should not try to predict what the hell is going to happen. First, I can drive again. Yeah, but that was not my last visit to see him. The man explained to me today that he follows his cancer patients for at least one-year post-surgery. I also got the result on the Assays. Both were negative, so my hope that maybe we could be able to go hormonal therapy is shot down the tubes, or up the tubes or whichever damn way they go.

It's amazing how my mood has changed over the last hour. When I was writing this letter to you, I was feeling down, then as I wrote I started to feel better, almost as good as having you here, started loosening up. Now I feel like shit again. But I will turn it around. At least I don't have to depend on anyone to drive me around.

Now in case you're wondering if I have lost my mind completely and think the worst is over, no. I am aware that what lies ahead may be a tad shaky, but I'm trying to maintain a positive attitude. I have heard all sorts of horror stories about Chemotherapy and what it is going to do to my body and my life, and it is important for me to play the negative aspects down as much as I can in an attempt to give my mind a chance to combat the side effects and turn it around. In addition, I am also aware that how I feel can and will change from day to day. I think this is the hardest part for Marty to grasp. Somedays I feel strong and able to do just about anything I want, and somedays, I don't want to get out of bed. And I think Marty sees it as a steady progression. Once I can do something again, then I'm okay for that thing. But I swear, somedays especially when it's cold, it feels like my armpit is trying to draw up into my chin.

It's also difficult for me to deal with being dependent on Marty economically. I've never tripped or perhaps I should say tripped much over the fact that she earned more money than I, but this latest situation is not at all acceptable. I think it's what was the final push to get me into this room. I think my fear of being kept overrode my fear of failure. As soon as I get a sense of how much effect the chemo has on me and for how long, I will try to set up a schedule of readings, lectures to earn some bread. Who knows, maybe I'll remember how to write and create something that I can sell too.

I'm supposed to go to Antioch College on the 1st, 2nd, and 3rd of February.[86] It's my bi-annual trip. Strangely about every two years I get a call from someone to come out there and do a reading. Normally it's quite enjoyable, because the campus has its own motel, which means no sharing anyone's home and I'm usually there in winter and get to see snow. This year, I'm a little nervous. This will be my first reading since the surgery, and I am more than a little nervous. It's strange. It's not like I walk around thinking about the fact that my breast is gone, but I'll pass a mirror in the house and noticed that the shape is different and then I become self-conscious. I'm assuming that this will pass at some point. And then again, maybe it won't.[87] It took me over 30 years to realize that I was not ugly. Damn the things we must survive to survive.

Also have another question for you. When you were here in February, you suggested that I make contact with Cheryl Clarke. Why?

Now, how did Cheryl Clarke jump up into the middle of this letter? Much too convoluted to retrace the process.

---

[86] In Ohio.

[87] Parker did become comfortable with her body. In the Epilogue to the reprint edition of *Movement in Black* (Firebrand Books, 1999), Marty Dunham wrote, "She left her pillow-like prosthesis on the dashboard of my truck at Stanford University on her way to a reading with Audre Lorde after I assured her that if it didn't make her more comfortable, she needn't wear it to make other people feel more comfortable. She never wore it again."

Sister love, I must thank you again for having Nancy send your manuscript to me.[88] It's amazing to me how you are world renowned as a poet, women falling all over themselves to get next to you, and I always feel closer to you through your prose. There's a vulnerability there that makes me want to gather you in my arms and hold you. I think it is easier for me to read the prose and simply feel. I get caught up reading your poetry much in the same way that I get caught up in reading James Baldwin. I tend to want to study it. Is this weird or what? Audre, don't read this wrong. It just occurs to me that someone could take this all wrong. However I am trusting that you know me well enough to get my drift.

As I told you on the phone, I was quite pleased to see your article in *Essence*.[89] One because those folks need to be hearing from you chile and two because I got to see this great photo of Diva Lorde in residence in the islands.[90] I can almost feel the sun myself. You must tell me all about your home now. Having been there for a quick minute, I'm really excited because this means I may be able to see you strolling around, Honey. Have to tell you chile that the rain forest blew my little southern USA mind. One second it's dry; next second it's raining and hard. Intense.

What is she not saying? I admit your courage. I don't know that I could take myself to another country, not know the language and turn myself over to anyone for anything. Hell I don't know if I could handle it if I was fluent in twenty languages and we're not talking some nationalistic nonsense here. I would be scared shitless. They made me cry in the train

---

[88]Nancy Bereano from Firebrand Books sent the manuscript pages to *A Burst of Light*.

[89]An excerpt from *A Burst of Light* appeared in the January 1988 issue of *Essence*.

[90]The excerpt featured a photograph of Lorde sitting on the beach in Saint Croix, Virgin Islands.

station in Paris and you know crying is not easy for me. In fact it is major trauma. I'm still waiting on my first good cry behind this crap. So far I managed 5 minutes when the pain hit and wouldn't go away because I said so. Freak Out.

Well love, I am about mid way down page six. Still undone, but I'm tired and need to stop. Please answer this letter; I need to hear from you. I have some major concerns about what this will do to my relationship with my lover, but I'm too tired to get into this now.

Define "processed foods." Marty and I are debating milk and canned tomatoes. Take care. I love you.

Pat

February 6, 1988

Dear Pat,

I put the letterhead on just to show off—how do you like it? Not only have I become computer literate (are you ready for this language) but even computer artistic! You see? If we had modern telephone hookups we could communicate directly screen to screen... Tomorrow the stars... but everything is so speeded up anyway, it feels like a piece of me is always moving in one and a quarter time to everyone else's one. Do you feel like that? And then other times for the instant you don't want it's slow motion to forever.

Listen, love, it's not like being in a relationship with someone younger than myself although you are—it's like being in a relationship with a beloved part of my own self. It's always been so difficult to love you from afar, and so costly to come in close, I put a lot of the stuff I learned about you and me into EYE TO EYE.[91]

I wish I had those unfinished letters, Patti, especially from Washington. I thought about you all a lot that weekend, sitting up in the Berlin cold, and then Yoli's letter saying she'd seen you and you were going back home to deal with a lump in your breast.[92] And then you called.

Whatever I have/know that is useful to you is yours. Most of all to hear from you when you speak, and believe you when you are silent.

So, my friend. As you see, they're all disgusting liars but we can use them, the doctors, I mean. Of course they don't tell

---

[91] "Eye to Eye: Black Women, Hatred, and Anger" is in *Sister Outsider* (Freedom, CA: The Crossing Press, 1984). Alexis De Veaux's discussion on the formation of Lorde's thinking about black women and anger is insightful and profound in *Warrior Poet* (290-295).

[92] Yoli is a long-time friend of Lorde.

you how much it's going to hurt and rush us out of the hospital while we're still euphoric from the damned anesthesia and then when the pain hits its- oh. I must have done something wrong! This spider up the wall routine standing close to the wall helps a LOT, and so does always elevating your elbow when you sit down, on the back of a chair, or even with your hand on your hip. It helps the lymph drain, and is a good habit to get into for lots of reasons. Like exercise, posture, muscular tension, etc.

Pat, I respect your decision about chemotherapy. ANY DECISION WE MAKE ABOUT OUR OWN BODIES AFTER CONSIDERING FACTS IS THE RIGHT DECISION! Our decisions do not kill us, they are you and me making a move for life. What kills us oh my sister is indecision and despair and turning ourselves over unheeding to any of those others- well-meaning and otherwise- you are always so sure THEY have the right answers. You are a survivor, Pat, and that battle on a physical level is now braided into our lives, but the war is not alien, now is it? You and me, we've been fighting all our lives.

Baby, five years is very long, and also very short. It's a real freakout to see it as a possible measure around all we want to do, isn't it? But it does get easier. I swear it. But it might get a little harder first.

It is one of the weapons of the motherfuckers- it's very useful for them having us see our disease as our failing. And the weaker sex at that! Check out Moishe Dayan in THE CANCER JOURNALS.[93] We're in a fucking war, baby, we're warriors and we got scars. None of us live for three hundred years, and we sure aren't going to be the first human beings to die of absolutely nothing! The fact we're writing these letters to each other is a triumph, Pat, I feel it and want you to feel

---

[93]Lorde's 1980 collection published by Aunt Lute Books and winner of the 1981 Gay Book of the Year from the American Library Association.

it too. You been doing what you came to do, sweetheart, and I think you changed the world. That's the kind of thing we both got to deal with. We've managed better than most, old girl. Cancer is not a punishment or a demerit. It's a fucking scourge that's getting worse because there are no real priorities for it's getting better because its very existence is big business as well as cost-intensive population control. You've got to root that one out, sweetheart. It has nothing to do with your failure. Because that feeling comes around a lot, and it's really destructive.

It's never been that simple, anyway Patti. BULLSHIT on it's our anger that caused our cancers! How much strontium-90 and racism have you absorbed today? I feel it's my anger that has helped keep me alive and what the hell else are we supposed to erect against their homophobic racist sexist poison - a submissive grin? WE WERE NEVER MEANT TO SURVIVE so under the circumstances, girlfriend, I think we've done pretty well, give or take a bad spell or two. Neither one of us is lying in the gutter gutted with no mind to be elsewhere, no work to do, and no one caring. And each one of us could have been and you know it and I know it, so let's not kid ourselves.

Of course none of that makes it any easier, and some days it's still like hitting the brick wall at 10 mph and no windshield. People don't know how to treat us. Give them time. Just make it perfectly clear that learning how is their responsibility, not yours. Anastasia and Cassidy you have to help deal with their feelings. Mattie from the Coop you do not.

The ups and downs and changes go on for a long time and that's very good. Marty is going to love you no matter what, goose, and as you get less tender and sore I guarantee that you will discover some interesting erotic possibilities that are bound to delight. More on this subject (one dear to my heart of course) in the next letter written in vanishing ink! Think of yourself as a one-breasted dahomeian amazon.[94] It helps counter balance the sense of loss. I'm glad you're getting into your body. She's different, and she's yours. Love her. It's a good thing you're going to Antioch. By the time you get this you will have returned. I hope it was a good experience. I remember going to Texas three weeks after my mastectomy and how it felt like a triumph, but VERY SHAKY. Good luck, girl.

Andrea has come and gone, so as I re-read your letter in this conversation it's freaky around time, because as I said I have this feeling so often of fluidity and swiftness as well as the variability of happenings. I thank you for the love you sent by her.

Adenocarcinoma is a tumor arising in the lining-tissue (inner or outer) of a gland. Slower-moving than lymphomas, which arise in the gland itself. Generically, has a better prognosis than Infiltrating Duct Carcinoma, the most common kind of breast cancer.

If you develop chemo reactions besides lethargy - which you will have to start learning how to make terms with anyway, (the hardest thing for me is still the lessening energies) - ask your doctor about vitamin C therapy massive doses of which seem to have good effects. You might also check out a holistic doctor because there are biologicals you can take in addition to chemo which counteract the side effects. I also want you to initiate a conversation with your chemotherapist about Adriamycin (if that is an ingredient in your 'soup' along with 5-fluor) and its effect on heart-muscle and whether that's anything you need to be concerned about.

About sister Cheryl. I said make contact because I hoped you two might have something to say to each other, plus since

---

[94] Dahomey was an African kingdom during the seventeenth, eighteenth, and nineteenth centuries in what is today Benin.

she's the editor of CONDITIONS.[95] I know she can use your input into her consciousness of what international is supposed to be, plus I have a weakness as you well remember believing that we can all save each other if we really try and I hear you say already didn't you learn nothing at all from the Felicia fiasco and when will you ever learn anyway.[96] Cheryl is just too far gone and I guess I just never will. Learn, that is. Darling child. WHAT HAPPENED.

I get your drift. We're both very vulnerable women, Pat, and the fact that we used our vulnerabilities to make our greatest strengths makes us powerful women, not failures. I love you.

And in case you have ever tried
To reach me
And I could not hear you
These words are in place
Of the dead air
Still
Between us[97]

And yes you do need to cry, but there's time enough for that. Just make sure that when it comes you know what it's about, because sometimes it will masquerade as fury or depression or the kicked fender or the state of the world, not to mention Cassidy's muddy boots. Or Doug Williams 5 consecutives possessions (Nah nah nah never thought I could change, huh?)

Europe was hard and terribly cold but very good in a lot of ways. The treatments worked very well for me, and I'm in

---

[95] *Conditions* was a journal that published from 1977 until 1990; Cheryl Clarke was a member of the editorial collective. For more information, see Julie R. Enszer, "'Fighting to Create and Maintain Our Own Black Women's Culture': *Conditions* Magazine, 1977-1990," *American Periodicals*, vol. 25, no. 2 (Fall 2015): 160-176.

[96] *Conditions* published two issues of international lesbian writing.

[97] Lorde is riffing on the poem "Sister, Morning Is a Time for Miracles" from *Chosen Poems* (New York: W. W. Norton, 1982).

better shape than I've been in a few years. I feel in a holding pattern now as far as metastases are concerned, and fighting hard to keep it that way for as long as possible. But Europe was good also because I could never have done it the way I did it without Gloria, and it also gave us a chance to re-examine our relationship in an atmosphere removed from the usual pressures and distortions yet at the same time not devoid of meaningful work.[98] And it was in Berlin that we first lived together for extended periods of time that beautiful terrible spring of 1984 when the doctors here were burying me and I was refusing to believe I had liver cancer and the Afro-German girls were blowing my mind to brilliant pieces. So this relatively calmer time gave us a chance to review that whole time in perspective and learn some very important things about ourselves and each other, as well as about being Black Women together in a White European world.[99]

I love living here in the Caribbean. It feels like I've come home, and St. Croix, where I have developed a community over the last seven years of coming in and out of it, feels particularly possible. But there are lots of culturally shocking changes that I'm learning to swing with. This is where I want to be, but the colonialism is yet another battlefront shaping up. As if I would have it any other way. The beaches, the sea, the coconuts, and the sun, as well as the power outages and the high prices. I wish you could come visit sometime. Remember it is a place you can come and be quiet.

It is deep and it is wonderful with Gloria, which doesn't mean it isn't sometimes rocky. It is still a hard time for Frances, who is putting her life together in a different way. I miss her,

---

[98]Gloria Joseph. Joseph and Lorde were in an intimate relationship at this point.

[99]*Audre Lorde: The Berlin Years 1984-1992*, directed by Dagmar Schultz (2012), examines Lorde's time in Germany and her interactions with Afro-German women.

but I am very happy, and pleased to know I deserve whatever I can harvest.[100]

You and Marty must talk honestly about your terrors and your expectations and your fears. Now. Not next year when it might be so much harder.

Processed foods are those with the life nuked or chemicalized out of them. When you come right down to it, cooking is processing, so use your own discretion. Anything with those weird sounding, alphabetical preserver chems are out. Canned tomatoes are very high in acid and not very good for you in general. Neither is milk, except unnuked goats' - but then that's me.

Dare I say answer soon? So much still to say, but I'm wearing out. Going to Anguilla for 2 weeks 2/14-29. Would love to have a letter when I come home. That number there will be 809-492-2351.

My love to you, and Marty, and Anastasia,
Audre

---

[100] Lorde's relationship with Frances Clayton officially ended when they sold the house in Staten Island in 1988 (*Warrior Poet*, 361).

March 12, 1988

And show off she did. Like how did you get that letterhead on that page? What kind of computer are you using and even more important, what word processing program are you using? I do have a modem. What I don't have is the software program to process it yet.

I decided here instead of going through your letter and answering your questions first, I would tell you what's been happening and what's on the brain this month and then go back to the letter.

When the NBLGC called you from Los Angeles, I was sitting in the audience.[101] It took all the control and reserves I have ever mustered in my life not to go up to that podium and snatch that phone from that woman, who had already pissed me off by introducing me as Pam Parker doing the morning session, and saying "Hi" to you. It felt so good to hear your voice even though you were actually talking to a crowd. I was a little worried when I got back to L.A. and found out you were not going to be there. You were the reason I decided to go for no goddamn money. Don't take that the wrong way, I had for the most part a good time. I got to see my sisters and niece and nephew. I met some interesting women, and didn't get too pissed at those folks, but the selling point for me was a chance to get to see you.

I don't understand the reasoning of the middle class. I go to this conference which is being held at a hotel as opposed to a campus or someplace. Now I can understand thinking hotel. It totally eliminates the need to arrange housing in the community, but it also prevents people who cannot afford to

---

[101] Ruth Waters and Phill Wilson founded the National Black Lesbian and Gay Leadership Forum. Originally a local organization, it addressed the need for black lesbians and gay men to organize nationally. The first conference was held in February 1988 in Los Angeles; Lorde addressed the attendees via telephone.

stay in hotels from attending the conference. The influence of the gay men was seen all over the place. There were no women, read my lips here - none, scheduled for the opening session. I wound up reading poetry for 10 minutes because Joe Beam didn't make it from Philadelphia.[102] Actually let me correct that. There was a slide show presented by a woman. Dr. somebody whose name I can't remember for shit which is unfortunate, because clearly she is someone to remember. The slide show was on Black folk who are or were gay. Audre, I had my mind blown all over the place. George Washington Carver. Lorraine Hansberry. I had to stop and go get my copy of the program from the conference and look up the woman's name, because she impressed me with her research. Dr. Sylvia Rhue. The slide show was called "Filling the Void."[103] You were in it. I must admit I took a little credit (privately of course) for the fact that you were in the show flashing back to our marathon conversation on Terrace Street.

While I'm on the subject of you appearing, let me get this question asked. When I was in Atlanta, a woman walked by me wearing a tee shirt with the following quote: "I have been a woman for a long time. Beware my smile. I am treacherous."[104] The punctuation is mine; the shirt was broken into four lines. The shirt acknowledged you as the author. I asked the woman where she got the shirt and she said what sounded like SUNY

---

[102] Joe Beam was a writer and literary activist during the 1980s. He edited *In the Life: A Black Gay Anthology* (Boston, MA: Alyson Books, 1986.) *Black Gay Genius: Answering Joseph Beam's Call*, edited by Steven G. Fullwood & Charles Stephens (New York: Vintage Entity Press, 2014) compiles excellent resources on Beam and the attention his work received prior to his death in 1988.

[103] Sylvia Rhue later became a documentary filmmaker, directing *All God's Children* about African-American families and homophobia as well as other documentaries.

[104] Lines from Lorde's poem "A Woman Speaks." Originally published in *The Black Unicorn* and included in *The Collected Poems of Audre Lorde* (New York: W. W. Norton, Inc., 1997).

Buffalo. Are you aware of these goodies and hopefully are getting royalties from their sale?

Now back to the conference. Great attention was paid to appearance. Fresh flowers, fairly decent food for a banquet. I heard one figure floating around of $8,000.00 for one banquet. And of course girl friend the folks was tabbed to the max. Phill Wilson in the course of two days and one night wore three tuxedos.[105] And they were handing out awards and plaques all over the place. So my question is how come the folks don't see it as a priority to pay their artists? I am so tired of benefits I could scream. In fact, I made a vow after this one and realizing that not only did I work for free, but I spent $100.00 that I couldn't afford on books, tee shirts, etc., that I will never again work for free for anybody. I don't care how Black, how Queer, how Womanly. NO money - no Parker.

The good side of this is the fact that I did get some information that I didn't have before; and if one of the people who approached me and asked about me during a reading in their town and took my cards actually came through and produced me for a sane fee then I will be delirious. Of course it's that type of thinking that gets me into these things in the first place.

Plus I got to spend three days looking at pretty Black folks. I swear there is something different and uniquely special about the way Black people move among each other, especially when there is less fear because of the support from numbers. I could sit for days upon end and just feel the flowing. And then knowing that the Black folks I was watching were gay. Actually though I suspect a part of the movement and it's specialness was the fact that the folks were gay and were not parading around in drag walks. Drag as in trying to be straight.

---

[105] In addition to founding the National Black Lesbian and Gay Leadership Forum, Phill Wilson is a distinguished HIV/AIDS activist. He is currently the Executive Director of the Black AIDS Institute.

Well, my child has just awoken from her nap and Marty is at the gym which I am playing hookey from because I wanted to clean up my studio and get this letter going; so I am going to close this for now and seize this time of just Anastasia and Pat and take her to the park. I shall return.

The trip to the park was wonderful. The sun was out and beautiful and Stasia delighted in showing off her skills on the monkey bars to me. Imagine back flips at 4 years old. It is now Sunday afternoon and I have about 10 minutes before I have to go to softball practice, so I decided to add to this letter.

Yesterday after we returned from the park, we had to go to Judy Grahn's for dinner. It was a wonderful meal of Greek salad and fresh pasta and salmon. Judy's new lover is a woman named Chris and I must say I find her far more attractive than Paula Gunn Allen.[106] Judy, by the way, has been very helpful since my diagnosis. She comes out approximately once a week and goes to the gym with me and we both flounder around in the pool and hang out in the sauna and whirlpool. She hasn't gotten bold enough to go to the racquetball court with me yet. It's actually been great. Last week I was so depressed that I started to call and cancel, but didn't. She managed to get me out of it; not by a bunch of false platitudes, but by understanding and listening. We've made plans to meet every Wednesday, as our schedules allow, to hang out. Who knows we might even learn how to swim in the process.

Would you believe it's been over two weeks since I started this letter? I have been doing a roller coaster ride of emotions and energy levels.

---

[106] Paula Gunn Allen was a poet, storyteller, and Native American cultural activist; she and Grahn were intimate partners.

May 10th

Well now it's been a hell of a long time since I started this letter and since I have yet to call your house without a busy signal I'm beginning to think that maybe there's something wrong with the phone system or I have the wrong number. Nobody can talk that much on the telephone. I've got 809-773-7891. Is that right?

Back to what I started to say - I've been emotionally up and down. I started out going great guns - the gym every day, eating well, not smoking. But over the last two months regressed back to all the same bad habits. And this is making me wonder what am I saying to myself. Is there some wish to die that I'm not facing? I don't think so, but I must admit I am beginning to wonder, especially after reading books like Siegel.[107]

Oh, before I forget. I did a reading at a local San Francisco bookstore and this woman walks up to me after the reading and wants to know why Audre Lorde and I have cancer. I didn't hit her, but I was a little more than pissed off at the implication of her question.

I have so many questions, and am getting a little frustrated (actually a lot frustrated) finding the answers. I have been trying to find a Black lesbian feminist therapist in this area. You would think this is easy, right? Not so. I've now gotten a couple of leads and we'll see where they pan out.

Before I forget, someone I don't remember who told me you are coming to the Bay Area for a reading during the summer. Is this true and if so when?

I did a reading at Stanford and this woman comes up to me; she says she's a friend of Beth's, so I took her name and

---

[107] Bernie Siegel's *Love, Medicine, and Miracles*, published in 1986, explores how patients can eliminate stress to promote healing.

number to send to you so you can pass it on. Her name is Erin Carlston, c/c Modern Thought & Literature, Stanford University, Stanford CA. 94305.

Adriamycin is not one of my soups, although it tends to create problems with heart patients who have problems with the heart itself as opposed to the arteries, which is where I ran into trouble.

Chemo is moving along o.k. I have had to work a little harder on my mind going in, because I started getting nauseous just thinking about my next appointment, but the last appointment I was able to leave go to the gym and play racquetball and go out that night and pitch a softball game, but I was a tired little puppy that next day, but a very proud little tired puppy.

Listen, I am so happy about your change of residence. Whenever I visualize you in that setting, I can't help but smile. The idea of that warm sun and beautiful blue water surrounding you makes me feel good. I know just enough about the U.S. Virgin Islands to realize that you are not in a paradise, and I hope the folks are ready for you. I still find it incredible that governments have the audacity to sell islands of people.

I have a friend from Puerto Rico who is on an education campaign about the destruction of the rain forest in her country. Is that happening there?

But back to you, I don't know Gloria, but I love her because you do. I realized after you told me about her, that I was very happy for you, but also feeling sad for Frances. I wanted to write Frances, but then I realized that I have actually met Frances one time in my life and my feelings for her were directly related to the fact that she loved you. So, I didn't think that a letter from me would have done her any good.

The trip to Antioch was wonderful and scary. I did a good job. They had arranged for me to have a massage and that was a little strange at first, but very helpful to me. I wrote a poem about the experience and when I get the kinks out I'll send it to you.

Since Antioch, I went to Xavier University to Cincinnati and next week I go to Ohio State. I don't know what the attraction for me is in Ohio, but as Willyce Kim says "take the money and run, honey."[108] I called you several times while I was in Ohio, but was unable to reach you.

If I'm ever able to put a couple of these readings back to back so that the money I earn isn't going straight to bills, I plan to come and see you.

Marty and Anastasia are both doing fine. Marty was a wreck for while between trying to take care of me and Stasia and starting a new job. When I came back from Ohio the second time she went straight to bed for a week with a virus that has been tearing up the Bay Area. Stasia was sick with the same virus for two weeks. Right now everybody is healthy.

I'm enclosing an article from "People" magazine. Have you any information on this case?[109] If so, let me know. Also do you have a VCR in your house? If the answer is yes, let me know what format. From time to time, I see shows on the tube and think that you might want to check them out. Last night PBS did a show on racism on college campuses. I was not aware of the rapid growth of madness. So, let me know if you have a machine and what kinds of things you might be interested in seeing.

---

[108] Willyce Kim is a Bay Area lesbian poet; she was a member of the Women's Press Collective, which published her chapbook, *Eating Artichokes*, and one of Parker's ex-lovers. Kim also published the poetry collection *Under the Rolling Sky* (1976), and two novels, *Dancer Dawkins and the California Kid* (Boston: Alyson Publications, Inc., 1985) and *Dead Heat* (Boston: Alyson Publications, Inc., 1988).

[109] The enclosed articles seems to be lost and not preserved in the archive.

I have the Super Bowl on tape, but I'll not send that, cause I know somebody must have told you Doug Willams' name.[110]

I'm going to let this letter go. Write me; let me know how and what you're doing. I'll try and get my next letter off sooner.

I love you.
Bye,
Pat

---

[110] Doug Williams was the first African-American quarterback to lead a team to victory in the Super Bowl. Williams was the quarterback for the Washington Redskins who defeated the Denver Broncos in Super Bowl XXII on January 31, 1988.

[October 1988][111]

Dear dear Pat,

This was going to be a long letter & it will be but drama got too intense. Gloria and I are in Hawaii for reading and relaxation (!) and this island has been so unexpectedly reassuring- the Volcano and the new/old earth mingling- Baby we can't help but be right- we echo Pele, the goddess who lives in the center. I'm reading at Stanford 11/9, maybe coming to SF 11/10 for NPR interview at 12:00- but out for Barbados at 10 PM 11/10. Any chance we can get together that day? I will call you when I get in 11/7 or 11/8 or... I look forward to our sitting down together A LOT.

Love, Audre

---

[111] This date is inferred from accounts of Lorde's travel in *Warrior Poet*.

September 8, 1988

Audre love,

This is not a piece of paper, but my arm extending across all the damn miles between us to hold you and hug you with all the strength, we have had to gain from the pain.

This is my hand reaching inside you to feel the hole that is there.

Right now I feel betrayed by words; there is nothing I can say that says what I feel.

September 9, 1988

I just got off the phone with you, so maybe now I can get this done. You say you want to know what is going on with me and I say I want to know what's going on with you. It feels like I'm just talking about me and that's not what I want.

So now I'll spend the next few pages talking about me. By now, hopefully, you've received a copy of Joan Larkin and Carl Morse's anthology.[112] In the dialogue between the two, we are given credit for spurring the renaissance of black gay writers and while I am pleased that at least that is acknowledged, I know that our work has touched a whole lot of other folks as well. Will I learn to just take what is given and not always question? I doubt it.

Changing gears here. Thank you. I did receive the copy of "A Burst of Light", and the money tucked in its pages.[113] I almost blew it. The postman did not deliver the book, but brought out one of those "pick this up at the office" slips. I have stopped

---

[112] Joan Larkin and Carl Morse, *Gay and Lesbian Poetry in Our Time* (New York: St. Martin's Press, 1988).

[113] Audre Lorde, *A Burst of Light* (Ithaca, NY: Firebrand Books, 1988).

picking those up, because usually it's a collection agency. Then I remember in our last phone conversation that you said, you were sending me a copy. So, I went down and Lo and behold, it was a missile of wisdom. I also realized that you might have misunderstood me. You asked me if I had read "A Burst of Light" and I said "no." What I meant was that I had not read the book. I did read the essay in manuscript form. Nancy Bereano sent me a copy. And for the life of me, I cannot remember what we were talking about when the question came up.

I was so glad to see the interview with Susan Leigh Star.[114] I was feeling quite isolated and alone since "Bar Conversation."[115] A few women have approached me and damn near whispered that they were glad I did the poem, but for the most part it has been silence.

As I read the book, it hit me again, what I have always known, that you are indeed a gutsy woman. Your speech at Medgar Evers was both so needed and courageous.[116] And "Apartheid USA" was right on time.[117] I have been bothered by what I call "white folks ability to only deal with one problem at a time." Actually it's not so much dealing with one thing at a time as it is, the ability to convince oneself that a particular problem has been adequately dealt with.

I am so tired of hearing how better off Black people in this country are. It blows my mind when the government comes out with a report showing that more and more Blacks

---

[114]Susan Leigh Star, "Sadomasochism: Not about Condemnation An Interview with Audre Lorde," appears in *A Burst of Light* and also in a slightly different form in *Against Sadomasochism: A Radical Feminist Analysis*, edited by Robin Ruth Linden, Darlene R. Pagano, Diana E. H. Russell, and Susan Leigh Star (San Francisco: Frog in the Well, 1982).

[115]Parker's poem, "Bar Conversation," is included in *The Complete Works of Pat Parker*.

[116]"I Am Your Sister: Black Women Organizing Across Sexualities" in *A Burst of Light*.

[117]Another essay in *A Burst of Light*.

and Hispanics are falling below the poverty line (which is in itself a joke) and in the same breath proceeds to say, that the report is good and the economy is up.

Feelings – so difficult to write about what is being felt. I just completed the nine week course at the Cancer Support and the Education Center in Menlo Park. Thank you again, Audre Lorde. One of things that becomes most apparent to me is how I smash down feelings and even refuse to write about them in my journal.

One of the things they do at the Center is to introduce you to the little girl in yourself. I met little Patty Parker and she is one frightened angry child. And a great part of that anger is at Pat Parker. I've realized that I have allowed myself to accept the myth of "strong Black woman" so much that I am actually afraid when the child in me appears. I think one of the most impressive things to me about "A Burst of Light" is your ability to talk about your fears in a real sense.

I have a new studio. Remember the room you slept in when you were here? Marty gave it to me in an effort to get me out of my rut. I think, in fact I know, for a while there I had given up; the ritual of doctors and tests, and my whole life seeming to be revolving around them, plus I think fear brought me to a complete stop.

I verbalized that I need a break; but I think in reality I was trying to direct my way of dying. I did everything my cardiologist told me not to do. On some subconscious level, I decided that I would rather die of a heart attack than cancer. I think I'm passed that now. I started the process all over again of trying to get the best that is in me out.

But Lorde child, as you know, it is a pain. I hate the question marks that chemotherapy puts into my life. How will I feel after this treatment? Will I have the energy to do what I need to do?

My sisters came up to visit around the time of my last treatment. When I came home, they had to wash off their accents of perfume and lotion, because the smells were making me sick. Now, what kind of shit is that? One of the most gorgeous things about Black woman for me has always been our scents.

I think what's frustrating here is that the cumulative effects of the chemo is making me weaker and that both frightens and angers me. In the beginning, I visualized and meditated it was really no problem for me at all. As I get more problems, I start doubting the effects of the visualization and meditation. If it's working, then why am I nauseous and tired? And, yes, I know about marijuana and nausea.

Oh! Good news for a change. There was a benefit for me, put on by this woman, Haley. She's a booking agent for some of the performers in the area. She got a whole ton of people to perform, and local businesses to donate to an auction, and so we were able to raise the rest of the money for me to go to Menlo Park. The show was eight hours long. Audre, I have never seen anything like it. There were people there Sharon Isabell, who hadn't done a reading for 8 years, and Willyce Kim, and Judy Grahn.[118] And musicians that I have worked with and some folks who were just being born when I started. There was food donated by local delis, and the preparation and serving, and cocktail waitressing, staffing of the raffle booths, etc. was all done by the members of the two softball teams I play on.

It was so bizarre to be sitting in a room and having people say what my work has meant to them. It was overwhelming at times, and I just wanted to run out of the room, but at the same time, it gave me validation for the choices I have made, and right now I can use all the validation I can get. Sometimes,

---

[118]Sharon Isabell (May 1, 1942-July 7, 2003) was the author of *Yesterday's Lessons* (Oakland, CA: Women's Press Collective, 1974); see note 107 on Willyce Kim; Judy Grahn continues to write and publish poetry, lesbian-feminist theory, and fiction.

when I get totally depressed, I play portions of the tapes from that night. Haley gave me copies of the entire show.

September 10th

I had to stop yesterday. Judy came over to go to the gym with me. I was ready to call her and give her hell. She's cancelled out for the last two months, and I do need that push to keep going. Judy told me that she saw you in Canada. I'm sorry about that; I know she put you in an awkward position. I never got to see her before she left, after our conversation. So if it will make things easier, I cannot come to see you in St. Croix.

I finally found out yesterday, why Judy has been being so flaky. We have been swimming at the gym; Judy has a fear of water and was progressing well, but she went down to San Diego and slipped and fell into a pool and that set her back to the beginning. Yesterday, she was able to get back into the pool, but was only able to stay in about five minutes.

Yesterday my little girl started kindergarten. Audre, you should have seen her. She was so full of herself. She's in an alternative program called the "Apple Project." It was recommended to us by the director of her pre-school, because she felt Stasia was too advanced for regular kindergarten. If it sounds like I'm bragging, I am. The kid is so bright and energetic.

Her pre-school had this project where the parents came in and described their work to the kids. So Marty went in and told them about roofing, and I went in and told them about writing and actually had them writing poems. They loved it and I was pleased. I even wore a dress, which Stasia decided was "the most beautiful dress in the world".

I went to Luisah Teish and had a reading done.[119] Was pretty positive, that afternoon when I came home I received

---

[119] In addition to her book *Jambalaya*, Teish offered divination readings.

a call from my doctor. My liver scan was suspect, so I had to go get a Cat scan. I was sweating bullets, and so pissed off. I couldn't believe that this would turn so fast on me. It turned out to be a cyst, they think.

Oh, in the closing session of the Cancer Center, one of the staff said, "how gutsy she thought I was that I don't wear a prosthesis." So I am going to send her a copy of "The Cancer Journal". As a part of the packet, that they give out, they include Bernie Siegel's and Carl Simonton's books.[120] Maybe after she reads yours; they will think about including it. Cross your fingers. If they go for it; it would mean hundreds of books per year.

Enough about me. What about you? I was worried and hurt when you didn't answer my last letter, but given what's been going on in your life it makes sense. So, how about a postcard when you can't write, just to let me know you're o.k.? I think about you often and talk to you a lot. I love you.

Please let me know what your schedule is going to be in November. Try and plan some time for us if at all possible. Give my regards to Gloria; she was so cute the other day talking to me until you got to another phone. FOUR PHONES!

Take care,
Love,
Pat

---

[120]Like Bernie Siegel's *Love, Medicine, and Miracles,* Carl Simonton's *Getting Well Again* (1978) outlined a "will to live" approach to cancer care and survival.

[1988 Christmas/Kwanza Card][121]

[printed inside:]

Wishing you Caribbean Christmas cheer
and joy and peace for the new year

[handwritten:]

Dear Pat, Marty, and Stasia,

I think of you all with love, and hope this coming new year will be a fruitful, open one for you and those you love! It was <u>very special</u> seeing you this fall!

Audre

---

[121] A handmade holiday card.

Pat Parker died on June 17, 1989
at the age of forty-five.

[From: Audre Lorde
A2 Judith's Fancy
Christiansted, St. Croix
U.S. Virgin Islands 00820

To: Marty Dunham][122]

Dear dear Marty,

I am so happy to hear from you! I've been wondering so often in these past terrible months how you and Stasia are, and what's happening!

Hugo was devastating, but we're getting back on our feet—exuberantly came back 12/17—3 months to the day after, & we are getting our roof put on right now & the glass finally replaced, and expect the phones by March. Gloria's fine, and I'm doing pretty well—have started infusion treatments here again because there are two new tumors in my liver, but the old ones are shrunk and I am confident I can beat it again. But if not, I'm living the life I choose.

I can't tell you Marty what it means to me to have the necklace from Pat—the reality of its power & that she thought of me. I loved her so much, Marty, and I feel her with me smiling so often. I asked my mom & her & Gloria's mom to help us, that terrible 13 hrs while Hugo mashed up our island & we cowered in a corner listening to the house breaking up around us. (And they did, too!) We're alive!

Sweetheart, I am so happy you are moving on with your life. I know that doesn't mean you don't still mourn Pat sometimes, but the best memorial to someone we love who is gone is to live fully and richly with whatever that person gave us! I know that to the depth of my being, and I want

---

[122]Handwritten notecard with addresses from the envelope.

you to know it too, because Patty would have wanted the best for you & Stasia. She loved you both, deeply, and when I promised her I would be whatever you needed me to be after she was gone (in our last telephone conversation) I meant it. Whatever.

If Kathleen is a good person and is good for you and Stasia, Pat would smile and bless you both and I sure do too. And don't you even listen for a moment to any meanness to the contrary!

You are a good woman, Marty, and I know what you gave Patty and how much you loved her, and also how very hard it sometimes was! And you deserve everything good out of life you ever find, for your devotion and your loyalty & your strength! There! I said it & I'm glad!

You tell Kathleen she's running with the Best, and hug Stasia for me. Tell her I'm coming out there again one of these days & we're gonna make some more house together!

Marty, sweetie, please remember I'm always here for you, not to intrude but to support, however you may need me.

Stay sweet!
Love Audre

P.S. Send me a photo of you and Stasia

St Croix
1-22-90

4/5/ POST HUGO

Audre Lorde died on November 17, 1992
at the age of fifty-eight.

Editor Note

When I first met Marty Dunham face to face (we had been corresponding via email for a while), she told me about the letters between Pat Parker and Audre Lorde. She said it was a beautiful correspondence and that selections from the letters had been read at a few tribute events to Parker and Lorde. I was intrigued. She did not have copies for me to read at that time. Two years later, I returned to the San Francisco Bay area to help Marty prepare Parker's papers for the Schlesinger Library and to do research to prepare *The Complete Works of Pat Parker*. One of the first things I did was read these letters. They were magical. Enchanting. Mesmerizing. These letters present an opportunity for readers to glimpse into the hearts and minds of two extraordinarily talented poets and writers. It has been only pleasure to spend time with these letters and edit them into this book.

Parker and Lorde met first in 1969 when Lorde was on a book tour on the West Coast. Wendy Cadden, a graphic artist and member of the Women's Press Collective, introduced the two women. Lorde was thirty-five years old (born February 18, 1934), and Parker was twenty-five (born January 20, 1944). The twenty-six letters of this extant correspondence (plus the final, twenty-seventh letter from Lorde to Marty Dunham) begins five years later in October 1974 after another visit by Lorde to the West Coast. The twenty-year friendship of Parker and Lorde, until Parker's death, covers the most productive years of their poetic and intellectual production.

One indication of the strength of their friendship is the dedication of works to one another. Parker's poem "For Audre" (*The Complete Works of Pat Parker*, 177) captures the vibrancy of the friendship between the two. Lorde dedicated her final collection, *The Marvelous Arithmetics of Distance*, published posthumously in 1993, to Parker with these words: "To My Sister Pat Parker, Poet and Comrade-in-Arms In Memoriam." The collection includes the poem "Girlfriend" which also captures some of their banter and the significance of the relationship for Lorde. These poems and letters hint at the rich friendship between these two poets.

A few notes on the text:

- Spelling errors have been silently corrected for ease of reading.
- Commas and other punctuation have been inserted and changed for reading convenience and are not noted.
- Footnotes to provide more information and to clarify various references for contemporary readers; they are designed to invite readers to explore the worlds and works of Parker and Lorde further and not distract from the words of Parker and Lorde.
- Pat Parker's papers, including copies of these letters, are housed at Arthur and Elizabeth Schlesinger Library on the History of Women in America, Radcliffe Institute for Advanced Study, Harvard University.
- Audre Lorde's papers, including copies of these letters, are housed at the Spelman College Archives.

Acknowledgements

I am grateful to Anastasia Dunham-Parker-Brady, Pat Parker's heir, and to Elizabeth Lorde-Rollins and Jonathan Rollins, Audre Lorde's heirs, for permissions for this project.

Martha Dunham has been an extraordinary advocate for this project as well as *The Complete Works of Pat Parker*; thank you, Marty for all of your time, attention, and generosity. Thank you to *Sinister Wisdom* interns who helped create the manuscript copy of the text. Thank you to the archivists who steward Parker and Lorde: Holly Smith at Spelman College and Kathryn Jacob at the Schlesinger. Thank you to attentive readers of the manuscript copy of this book: Cheryl Clarke, Maxx Bauman, Sara Gregory, and Zane DeZeeuw.

Thank you to the board and subscribers to *Sinister Wisdom* for supporting this work. Thank you to Lawrence Schimel of A Midsummer Night's Press for partnering to produce the book. As always, thank you to my beloved wife, Kim, not a reader of poetry but lover of a poet and all she does.

All errors are, of course, my own.

Julie R. Enszer, PhD
February 2018

Audre Lorde
Partial Bibliography

Poetry Collections

The First Cities (New York: Poets Press, 1968).

Cables to Rage (Detroit: Broadside Press, 1970).

From a Land Where Other People Live
(Detroit: Broadside Press, 1973).

The New York Head Shop and Museum
(Detroit: Broadside Press, 1974).

Coal (New York: W. W. Norton, 1976).

Between Our Selves (Point Reyes: Eidolon, 1976).

The Black Unicorn (New York: W. W. Norton, 1978).

Chosen Poems Old and New
(New York: W. W. Norton, 1982).

Our Dead Behind Us (New York: W. W. Norton, 1986).

Undersong: Chosen Poems Old and New
(New York: W. W. Norton, 1992).

The Marvelous Arithmetics of Distance
(New York: W. W. Norton, 1993).

The Collected Poems of Audre Lorde
(New York: W. W. Norton, 1997).

Prose Collections

The Cancer Journals
(San Francisco: Spinsters Ink, 1980).

Zami: A New Spelling of My Name
(Berkeley: Crossing Press, 1982).

Sister Outsider (Berkeley: Crossing Press, 1984).

A Burst of Light (Ithaca: Firebrand Books, 1988).

Need: A Chorale for Black Women Voices
(Brooklyn: Women of Color Press, 1990).

Pat Parker
Partial Bibliography

Poetry Collections

Movement in Black
(Oakland, California: Diana Press, 1978;
Trumansburg, New York: Crossing Press, 1983;
Ithaca, New York: Firebrand Books, 1990, 1999).

Jonestown & Other Madness
(Ithaca, New York: Firebrand Books 1985).

Womanslaughter
(Oakland, California: Diana Press, 1978).

Pit Stop
(Oakland, California: Women's Press Collective, 1974, 1975).

Child of Myself
(San Lorenzo, California: Shameless Hussy Press, 1971; Oakland, California: Women's Press Collective, 1972, 1974).

The Complete Works of Pat Parker
(Dover, FL: A Midsummer Night's Press and Sinister Wisdom, 2016).